Integrated Clinical Science

Endocrinology

Edited by
CRW Edwards, MD, FRCP (Lond, Edin)

Professor of Clinical Medicine, University of Edinburgh.
Chairman, Department of Medicine, Western General Hospital, Edinburgh

Series Editor
George P McNicol, MD, PhD, FRCP
(Lond, Edin, Glasg), FRCPath, Hon FACP

Principal and Vice Chancellor, University of Aberdeen. Lately Professor of Medicine, The University of Leeds, and Head, The University Department of Medicine, The General Infirmary, Leeds

William Heinemann Medical Books Ltd
London

First published 1986
© 1986 William Heinemann Medical
   Books Ltd, 23 Bedford Square,
   London WC1B 3HH

ISBN 0–433–16607–X

Printed and bound in Great Britain by the
Alden Press, Oxford

Contents

Acknowledgements

I would like to thank the Medical College of St Bartholomew's Hospital for permission to redraw Figs. 2.1, 2.2, 2.3, 2.9, 2.10 and 2.22 from original drawings by Bryony Carfrae. Figures 2.18 and 2.20 were originally published by Chapman & Hall in *Management of Pituitary Disease*, edited by Paul Belchetz.

I would like to thank Dr Eva Kohner of the Hammersmith Hospital, London for supplying the photographs for Fig. 8.49.

A number of figures have been redrawn from figures in the following publications:

Fig. 5.5:   Odell W.D. (1979). *Endocrinology* Vol. III (L. J. DeGroot, ed.), p. 1387. Grune & Stratton.

Fig. 8.2:   Orci L. (1982). *Diabetes*; **31**: 554.

Fig. 8.3:   Orci L. (1982). *Diabetes*; **31**: 557.

Fig. 8.5:   Bonner-Weir S., Orci L. (1982). *Diabetes*; **31**: 888.

Fig. 8.9:   Metz R. (1960). *Diabetes*; **9**: 92.

Fig. 8.12:   Gibby O.M., Hales C.N. (1983). *Br. Med. J.*; **286**: 922.

Fig. 8.20:   Woods S.C., Smith P.H., Porte D. Jr (1981). *Handbook of Diabetes Mellitus*, Vol. 3, p. 213. John Wiley & Sons.

Fig. 8.25:   Garber A.J., Cryer P.E. *et al.* (1976). *J. Clin. Invest.*; **58**: 7.

Fig. 8.26:   Baird J.D. (1974). *A Companion to Medical Studies*, Vol. 3, p. 77. Blackwell Scientific Publications Ltd.

Fig. 8.27:   Cudworth A.G., Wolf E. (1982). *Clinics in Endocrinology and Metabolism*, Vol. 11, p. 396. W.B. Saunders Co. Ltd.

Fig. 8.28:   *Ibid.*, p. 400.

Fig. 8.29:   Baird J.D. (1974). *A Companion to Medical Studies*, Vol. 3, p. 75. Blackwell Scientific Publications Ltd.

Fig. 8.30:   Baird J.D. (1973). *Symposium on Anorexia and Obesity*, No. 42, p. 85. Royal College of Physicians of Edinburgh.

Fig. 8.31:   Baird J.D. (1974). *A Companion to Medical Studies*, Vol. 3, p. 75. Blackwell Scientific Publications Ltd.

Fig. 8.33:   *Ibid.*, p. 75.

Fig. 8.36:   Baird J.D. (1980). *Symposium on Nutrition*, No. 53, p. 74. Royal College of Physicians of Edinburgh.

Fig. 8.40:   Baird J.D. (1974). *A Companion to Medical Studies*, Vol. 3, p. 89. Blackwell Scientific Publications Ltd.

Fig. 8.43:   Paisey R.B. (1980). *Diabetologia*; **9**: 92.

Fig. 8.48:   Trevor-Roper P.D. (1971). *Lecture Notes on Ophthalmoscopy*, 4th edn. Blackwell Scientific Publications Ltd.

Finally I would like to thank Clare Little for preparing the final artwork from the original rough sketches.

CRW Edwards

Preface

It is clearly desirable on educational grounds to adopt and teach a rational approach to the management of patients, whereby the basic scientific knowledge, the applied science and the art of clinical practice are brought together in an integrated way. Progress has been made in this direction, but after twenty-five years of good intentions, teaching in many medical schools is still split up into three large compartments, preclinical, paraclinical and clinical, and further subdivided on a disciplinary basis. Lip-service is paid to integration, but what emerges is often at best a coordinated rather than an integrated curriculum. Publication of the INTEGRATED CLINICAL SCIENCE series reflects the need felt in many quarters for a truly integrated textbook series, and is also intended as a stimulus to further reform of the curriculum.

The complete series will cover the core of clinical teaching, each volume dealing with a particular body system. Revision material in the basic sciences of anatomy, physiology, biochemistry and pharmacology is presented at the level of detail appropriate for Final MB examinations, and subsequently for rational clinical practice. Integration between the volumes ensures complete and consistent coverage of these areas, and similar principles govern the treatment of the clinical disciplines of medicine, surgery, pathology, microbiology, immunology and epidemiology.

The series is planned to give a reasoned rather than a purely descriptive account of clinical practice and its scientific basis. Clinical manifestations are described in relation to the disorders of structure and function which occur in a disease process. Illustrations are used extensively, and are an integral part of the text.

The editors for each volume, well-known as authorities and teachers in their fields, have been recruited from medical schools throughout the UK. Chapter contributors are even more widely distributed, and coordination between the volumes has been supervised by a distinguished team of specialists.

Each volume in the series represents a component in an overall plan of approach to clinical teaching. It is intended, nevertheless, that every volume should be self-sufficient as an account of its own subject area, and all the basic and clinical science with which an undergraduate could reasonably be expected to be familiar is presented in the appropriate volume. It is expected that, whether studied individually or as a series, the volume of INTEGRATED CLINICAL SCIENCE will meet a major need, assisting teachers and students to adopt a more rational and holistic approach in learning to care for the sick.

George P. McNicol
Series Editor

Contributors

KGMM Alberti
Professor of Medicine
The Medical School
Newcastle Upon Tyne

DC Anderson
Reader and Honorary
Consultant Physician
Hope Hospital
Manchester

JD Baird
Senior Lecturer and Honorary
Consultant Physician
Western General Hospital
Edinburgh

CRW Edwards
Professor of Clinical Medicine
Western General Hospital
Edinburgh

DA Heath
Reader and Honorary
Consultant Physician
Queen Elizabeth Hospital
Birmingham

WJ Jeffcoate
Consultant Physician
City Hospital
Nottingham

PL Padfield
Consultant Physician
Western General Hospital
Edinburgh

WMG Tunbridge
Consultant Physician
Newcastle General Hospital
Newcastle Upon Tyne

JAH Wass
Senior Lecturer and Honorary
Consultant Physician
St Bartholomew's Hospital
London

Advisory Editors

Professor AS Douglas
Department of Medicine, University of Aberdeen

Pathology: Professor CC Bird
Institute of Pathology
University of Leeds

Physiology: Professor PH Fentem
Department of Physiology and
Pharmacology
Nottingham University

Biochemistry: Dr RM Denton
Reader in Biochemistry
University of Bristol

Anatomy: Professor RL Holmes
Department of Anatomy
University of Leeds

Pharmacology: Professor AM Breckenridge
Department of Clinical
Pharmacology
Liverpool University

1

Introduction to the General Principles of Endocrinology

Few subjects in medicine have grown so dramatically as endocrinology. Advances in our understanding of the basic physiology underlying hormone secretion and action have rapidly led to better methods of investigating and treating pathophysiology. Conversely, the study of endocrine diseases has played a critical role in our appreciation of the complexity of normal endocrine function.

Hormones are defined as chemical messengers which coordinate the activities of different cells in multicellular organisms. However it has recently been appreciated that unicellular organisms such as the coliform bacillus, which has only one-thousandth of the DNA content of a human cell, are also capable of producing hormones. *E. Coli* has been shown to produce insulin, calcitonin, and a molecule similar to human chorionic gonadotrophin. This has been called an *autocrine* system (Fig. 1.1). As yet we know nothing of the uses to which these hormones are put.

The next evolutionary step was the development of an *isocrine* system in which non-specialised cells produce hormones which affect adjacent cells (Fig. 1.1). These hormones can be transferred either by simple diffusion or by conjugation of the cells such as occurs for *E. Coli*.

With increasing specialisation, certain types of cell emerged which had the ability to make specific hormones and, through them, to influence the function of surrounding cells. This, the *paracrine* system, is assuming major importance as more of these local hormone systems are discovered. A classic example is the organisation of the islet of Langerhans in the pancreas (p. 135). Four different types of cell have been identified in the human islet. The A cells secrete glucagon and form the outer rim of the cortex (Fig. 1.2). They make up 25% of the endocrine pancreas. In the

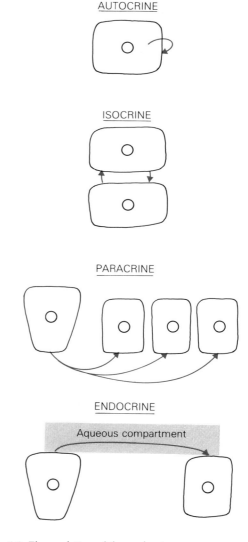

AUTOCRINE

ISOCRINE

PARACRINE

ENDOCRINE

Aqueous compartment

Fig. 1.1 *The evolution of the endocrine system.*

1

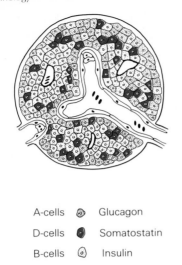

A-cells   Glucagon

D-cells   Somatostatin

B-cells   Insulin

Fig. 1.2 *Cell types in the pancreatic islet.*

ventral pancreas they are replaced by cells secreting pancreatic polypeptide. The insulin-secreting beta cells constitute 60% and are principally in the medulla. The D cells secreting somatostatin are situated between the A and the B cells. This intimate relationship is critical for the normal functioning of the islet. Somatostatin can inhibit the secretion of insulin and glucagon. These hormones in turn can alter the secretion of each other and also of somatostatin. Specialised techniques have demonstrated tight and gap junctions between these different types of cell (further details of this and of the control of insulin secretion are given in Chapter 8). All this suggests that the pancreatic islet acts as a syncytium.

The *endocrine* system was an inevitable consequence of the need for rapid communication between different parts of large multicellular organisms. Specialised cells release their products directly into an aqueous compartment such as the blood or cerebrospinal fluid and thus exert their effects at a distance from the site of secretion (Fig. 1.1).

DEVELOPMENT OF CLINICAL ENDOCRINOLOGY

The origins of clinical endocrinology go back into ancient history. Hippocrates included some important endocrine observations in his aphorisms. The medieval Chinese used seaweed in the treatment of iodine-deficient goitres. There was, however, little progress until about 200 years ago. In 1775 Percival Pott, a surgeon at St Bartholomew's Hospital, reported the case of a young woman with bilateral inguinal herniae. In repairing these he removed both ovaries and observed that following surgery her breasts atrophied and periods ceased. The importance of this observation was realised by John Davidge (1768–1829). He concluded that 'menstruation is attributable to a peculiar condition of the ovaries, serving as a source of excitement to the vessels of the womb'.

The science of experimental endocrinology was born in 1849. Professor Berthold from Göttingen carried out experiments on six young cocks (Fig. 1.3). Cocks A, B and C were two months old and D, E and F three months old. Cocks A and D were castrated and showed typical eunuchoid behaviour with atrophy of their wattle and comb. Cocks B and E had a bilateral orchidectomy but one testis was then put back into its normal position. These cocks developed as normal males. Cocks C and F had a bilateral orchidectomy. One testis from cock C was then placed in the peritoneal cavity of cock F and a testis from cock F in the normal position in cock C. Both cocks developed as normal males and the testes were found to be revascularised in their new sites. Berthold concluded that 'as the testes transplanted to a different place can no longer be connected with their original nerves. . . it follows that the consensus in question (i.e. the development of male behaviour) is conditioned by the secre-

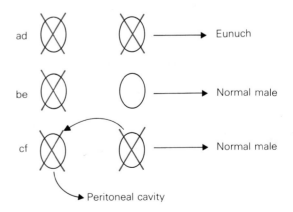

Fig. 1.3 *The birth of scientific endocrinology: experiments by Professor Berthold (1849).*

tion of the testes.' This paper is a model for any aspiring scientist in its brevity, experimental design and the clear-cut nature of the results and conclusions.

In 1855 Thomas Addison published his famous monograph on diseases of the suprarenal capsules. Addison's interest in skin diseases focused on the pigmentation of these patients and he coupled this with careful post-mortem examination which revealed the disease of the adrenal glands. The commonest adrenal disease was tuberculosis. The endocrine nature of this condition was not appreciated.

In 1895 Oliver and Schafer showed that extracts of the pituitary could elevate blood pressure, as could extracts of the adrenal. Howell (1898) then showed that the active principle in the pituitary resided in the posterior part of the gland. At the same time Tigerstedt and Bergman demonstrated that kidney extracts could raise blood pressure. The active principle was called renin. In 1902 Magnus and Schafer demonstrated the critical role of the posterior pituitary in the control of water balance. We now appreciate that the posterior pituitary principle, vasopressin, is not important in blood pressure control but is vital for fluid balance and is the antidiuretic hormone.

In 1904 Bayliss and Starling published their classic studies in which they showed that an extract of the duodenum boiled in dilute hydrochloric acid, neutralised, and injected into animals stimulated the flow of pancreatic juice. They proposed that a substance was produced by the duodenal epithelium in an inactive form which they called pro-secretin that was then converted by acid into the active compound secretin (Fig. 1.4). This concept of an inactive compound being produced that requires activation before release into the circulation is now known to be true for the products of many of the endocrine tissues.

W. B. Hardy proposed the name *hormone* (from the Greek 'to stir up') and this term was adopted by Starling (Fig. 1.5). Schafer, however, objected to this as some agents which produce depression or cessation of function were known to be produced in the endocrine glands. He suggested that these should be called *chalones* and that the term *autacoids* should be used to describe those specific organic substances formed by cells of one organ and passed from them into the circulation to produce effects upon other organs. These two terms, however, were never adopted but history has shown that Schafer's original concept was correct.

W. B. Hardy	— hormone	(ὅρμάω, to stir up)
E. Schäfer	— chalone	(χαλάω, to make slack)
	— autacoids	(ἁυτός, self: ἁκος, remedy)

Fig. 1.5 *The etymology of hormone, chalone and autacoids.*

Modern endocrinology evolved rapidly from these auspicious beginnings. Improvements in protein and steroid chemistry led to the isolation of a large number of hormones and eventually to the determination of their structures. Many of these have now been synthesised. This has greatly facilitated endocrine replacement therapy. Modern methods of hormone assay (principally radioimmunoassay, see p. 14) have transformed the assessment of endocrine function. This has in turn led to the introduction of sophisticated dynamic function tests. These are often critical in the assessment of endocrine reserve.

THE ROLE OF HORMONES

The products of endocrine glands subserve four major functions in the body. First, under basal conditions they

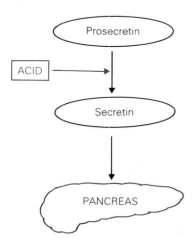

Fig. 1.4 *The activation of prosecretin by acid. Experiments by Bayliss and Starling in 1904.*

play a critical role in the maintenance of the so-called *milieu interieur*. Thus for example the concentration of salt in the body fluids is kept remarkably constant, principally by regulating the intake of water and the excretion of sodium and water by the kidney. A lack of aldosterone, the major salt-retaining hormone, will lead to a loss of salt and hence a low level of salt in the blood – depletional hyponatraemia (see Chapter 4). Oversecretion of the antidiuretic hormone (ADH) will lead to excessive conservation of water and a reduction of the blood salt concentration – dilutional hyponatraemia (see Chapter 7). Conversely, a failure of production of ADH will lead to excessive water loss by the kidney (diabetes insipidus) and hence hypernatraemia (see Chapter 2). Overproduction of aldosterone as by an aldosterone-secreting adrenal tumour will also elevate plasma sodium (Chapter 4). This contrasts with normal hormonal function, where the endocrine system, despite fluctuations in the external environment, keeps the level of critical substrates, enzymes and cofactors optimal for efficient metabolism.

Secondly, hormones play a vital part in the response of the organism to *stress*. This can take many forms such as starvation, infection, trauma or psychological pressures. Hormones such as adrenocorticotrophin (ACTH), growth hormone (GH) and prolactin are readily released in these circumstances and are thus often referred to as 'stress' hormones. Stress may also alter the metabolism of hormones. Thus thyroxine (T_4) instead of being metabolised to the much more biologically active hormone tri-iodothyronine (T_3) is converted to the biologically inactive reverse tri-iodothyronine (reverse T_3) (see Chapter 3).

The third major function of hormones is the *control of growth*. Growth hormone produced by the anterior pituitary stimulates the liver to synthesise a growth factor which then acts directly on the tissues. This effect then interacts with those of a number of other hormones such as thyroxine, insulin and sex steroids to produce the normal integrated pattern of growth (Chapters 2 and 8).

Finally hormones are essential for the *processes of reproduction*. They control libido, potency and fertility in the male and cyclical gonadal function and fertility in the female. *In utero* they are important for the development of the male genital ducts and external genitalia (Chapter 5).

THE STRUCTURE OF HORMONES

There are three main groups of hormones with different chemical structures. These are classified as being protein or peptide, steroid and amino acid. Examples of these are given in Table 1.1. With the exception of dopamine, all the hypothalamic and pituitary hormones come into the first category, as do the hormones originating from the pancreas and gut. If the protein contains a carbohydrate moiety it is referred to as a glycoprotein (Fig. 1.6). The *glycoprotein* hormones include luteinising hormone (LH), follicle stimulating hormone (FSH), human chorionic gonadotrophin (HCG) and thyroid stimulating hormone (TSH). These all share a common α subunit and have different β subunits. The *polypeptide* hormones are produced as part of a much larger precursor molecule which is then broken down to the smaller active hormone. For example, adrenocorticotrophic hormone (ACTH) is produced as part of pro-opiocortin which is then broken down to yield ACTH, β-lipotrophin (β-LPH) and an amino terminal sequence containing γ-melanocyte stimulating hormone (γ-MSH) (Fig. 1.7). ACTH itself contains 39 amino acids but only the first 24 are necessary for biological activity. Another example of a precursor hormone is proinsulin. This also is cleaved by intracellular proteolysis to yield insulin which has two chains linked by disulphide bonds (see Fig. 8.6, p 137). In proinsulin the two chains are linked by a connecting or C-peptide. This is released into the circulation at the same time as insulin and can be measured as an index of insulin secretion.

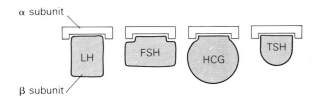

Fig. 1.6 *The structure of the glycoprotein hormones showing the common* α *subunit and the variable* β *subunit.*

Table 1.1

Classification of Hormones on Basis of their Chemical Structure

Protein and polypeptide	Origin	Steroid	Origin
Gonadotrophin-releasing hormone (GnRH)		Cortisol	
Thyrotrophin-releasing hormone (TRH)		Aldosterone	Adrenal cortex
Growth hormone release inhibitory hormone (GHRIH or somatostatin)	Hypothalamus	Corticosterone	
		Testosterone	Testis
Luteinising hormone (LH)		Dihydrotestosterone	Peripheral conversion
Follicle stimulating hormone (FSH)		Oestradiol (E_2)	Ovary
Prolactin		Progesterone	Ovary
Growth hormone (GH)		25-hydroxyvitamin D_3	Liver
Adrenocorticotrophin (ACTH)	Pituitary	1,25-dihydroxyvitamin D_3	Kidney
β-lipotrophin (β-LPH)			
Thyroid stimulating hormone (TSH)		*Amino acid and others*	
* Vasopressin (antidiuretic hormone ADH)		Thyroxine (T_4)	Thyroid
* Oxytocin		Tri-iodothyronine (T_3)	Thyroid and peripheral conversion
Parathyroid hormone (PTH)	Parathyroid	Adrenaline	Adrenal medulla
Calcitonin	Thyroid	Noradrenaline	Sympathetic nerves
Insulin	Pancreas	Dopamine	Hypothalamus
Glucagon	Pancreas	Melatonin	Pineal
Gastrin	Stomach		
Secretin	Duodenum		
Human chorionic gonadotrophin (HCG)	Placenta		

* Synthesised in hypothalamus but stored in posterior pituitary

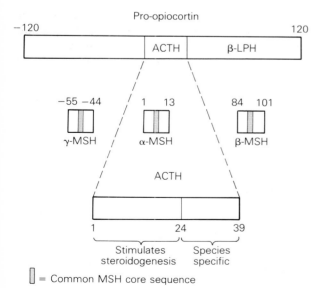

Fig. 1.7 *The structure of the ACTH and β-LPH precursor molecule, pro-opiocortin.*

The *steroid* hormones have as their basic ring structure the cyclopentanophenanthrene nucleus (Fig. 1.8). The major sources of steroids are the adrenal glands and the gonads. Some steroids, however, can be produced by peripheral conversion of a precursor in tissues such as fat or genital skin. The latter, for example, contains a 5α-reductase enzyme which converts testosterone, the major male hormone, to its more potent metabolite dihydrotestosterone. The D family of vitamins are also classified as steroid hormones and are referred to as secosteroids. In these compounds, the B ring of the steroid nucleus is open (Fig. 1.8). They also conform to the biological principle of being initially in the form of an inactive precursor which is then metabolised to an active product. In this case cholecalciferol (vitamin D_3) is converted by the liver to 25-OH-cholecalciferol, which is then in turn metabolised to the active compound 1,25-dihydroxy-cholecalciferol by the kidney (see Chapter 6).

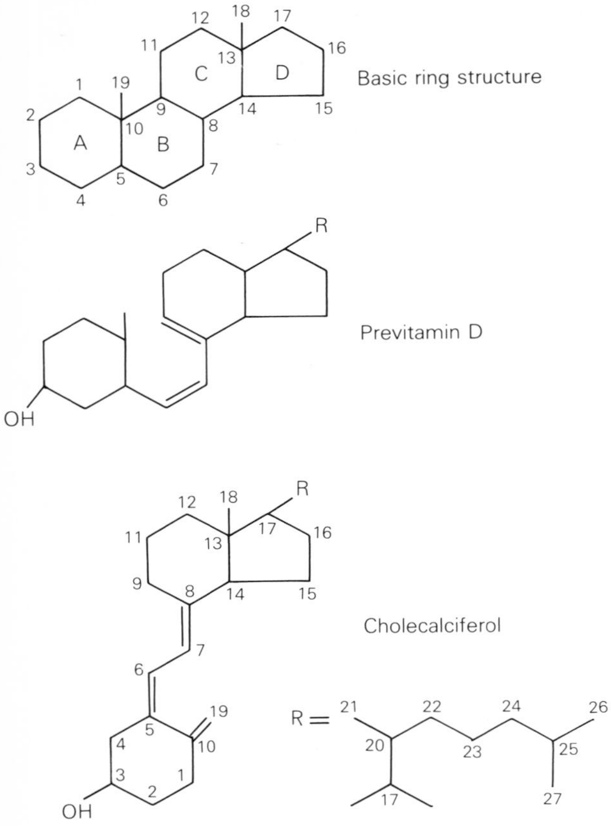

Fig. 1.8 *The structure of the steroid hormones.*

The structures of the amino acid and other hormones are shown in Chapters 3 and 7. Tyrosine is the basic substrate which can be iodinated and then coupled to another iodotyrosine to form thyroid hormone, or undergo a series of reactions catalysed by various enzymes to form dopamine, noradrenaline and adrenaline.

Biosynthesis of Hormones

The biological processes leading to the synthesis of a hormone can be classified on the basis of the structure

of the hormone. *Protein and polypeptide* hormone synthesis by endocrine cells depends on stimulation of DNA *transcription*. In this process the DNA acts as a template for the production of specific messenger (mRNA), ribosomal (rRNA) and transfer RNA (tRNA) molecules (Fig. 1.9). The DNA and its RNA transcripts contain the genetic code which determines the sequence of amino acids in the hormones to be synthesised. The amino acids are coded by groups of three bases called codons. There are 64 possible codons; of these, 61 code for amino acids and three act as signals to stop chain synthesis. As there are only 20 amino acids this means that many of them have more than one codon.

After leaving the nucleus the mRNA molecules migrate to the ribosomes on the rough endoplasmic reticulum. It is here that 'translation' takes place leading to protein synthesis. Many ribosomes can be involved in the translation of a single mRNA molecule. This collection of ribosomes is called a polysome (Fig. 1.9). The protein chains are formed from the amino to the carboxyl end (this involves reading the code from the 5' to the 3' direction).

The transfer RNA molecules consist of about 80 nucleotides and play a crucial role in transporting amino acids to the correct position on the mRNA template. Each tRNA has an amino acid attachment site and a template recognition site. Specific enzymes link particular amino acids to their own tRNA. This then has a three-base sequence (called an anticodon) which identifies the correct place on the template.

Protein synthesis is halted by termination codons. These lead to the production of factors which hydrolyse the bond between the polypeptide and the tRNA. The completed molecule is then transported to the Golgi apparatus where it is packaged for eventual export out of the cell by the process of exocytosis (Fig. 1.9).

In contrast to this process, *steroid* hormones are synthesised by a specific series of enzyme-catalysed reactions using cholesterol as substrate. This is either synthesised *de novo* within the cell or taken up by the cell via specific low density lipoprotein receptors. Cholesterol (27 carbon atoms) is the precursor of the five main types of steroid hormone; progestagens (C21), glucocorticoids (C21), mineralocorticoids (C21), androgens (C19) and oestrogens (C18). The steps leading to the formation of pregnenolone (a key

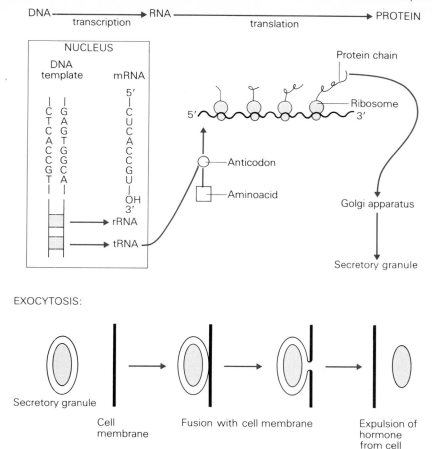

Fig. 1.9 *The biosynthesis of protein and polypeptide hormones and mechanism of hormone discharge from the cell by exocytosis.*

intermediate in steroid biosynthesis) in response to stimulation by adrenocorticotrophin (ACTH) of an adrenal cell are shown in Fig. 1.10. The activation of adenylate cyclase after the reaction of ACTH with a specific cell surface receptor leads to the production of cyclic AMP. This then activates a protein kinase cascade which results in increased transport of cholesterol into the mitochondrion, where side-chain cleavage occurs leading to the formation of pregnenolone. This process does not involve DNA transcription and hence inhibitors of this process such as actinomycin D do not inhibit it. Protein synthesis, however, is important and, if this is blocked by cycloheximide, steroidogenesis will not take place. The biosynthesis of thyroid hormones is detailed in Chapter 3 and of catecholamines in Chapter 7.

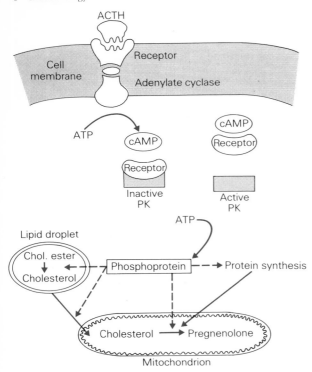

Fig. 1.10 *The biosynthesis of steroid hormones in response to stimulation of adrenal cell by ACTH.*

TRANSPORT OF HORMONES TO TARGET TISSUES

After hormones have been released from the specialised endocrine cells they need to be transported to their site of action. If this is to be on adjacent cells (i.e. a paracrine effect) then transport is usually by simple diffusion. When hormones are released into the blood, more complicated transport mechanisms are often used. Certain hormones, especially those with steroid and amino acid structures, have specific transport proteins. Such hormones circulate bound to these proteins which then protect them from metabolism and thus prolong their life in the circulation. The hormone-binding protein complex also acts as a reservoir of stored hormone. Thus circulating cortisol is almost all in the bound (biologically inactive) form (bound to cortisol-binding globulin-CBG), as is thyroxine (bound to thyroxine-binding globulin-TBG). These complexes then dissociate to produce the free (biologically active) hormones. The importance of these transport proteins is unclear; some individuals with apparently normal endocrine function have genetic defects resulting in an inability to synthesise a specific binding protein. Their clinical importance lies in the fact that most hormone assays measure total (i.e. bound and free) as opposed to the free hormone. This is mainly because of the technical difficulties in assaying the very low free hormone levels. If the level of the binding protein is altered this will change the total hormone level but, because of the feedback control systems, the free hormone level is unchanged. Oestrogen, for example, in the oral contraceptive pill will increase the level of thyroxine binding globulin and hence total thyroxine. A clinician unaware of this could make the mistake of diagnosing thyroid overactivity.

THE MECHANISMS OF ACTION OF HORMONES ON TARGET TISSUES

When considering how hormones produce their biological effects it is helpful to classify them into two groups – those that are water-soluble (the peptide hormones and the catecholamines) and those that are lipid-soluble (the steroids, the thyroid hormones, 1,25-dihydroxyvitamin D_3). The importance of this classification is that it divides hormones into those that cannot easily cross the phospholipid cell membrane (water-soluble) and those that can easily penetrate into the cell (lipid-soluble).

The water-soluble hormones have their main effect by reacting with specific receptors on the cell surface, as compared with the lipid-soluble hormones which usually bind to cytoplasmic receptors (Fig. 1.11). The water soluble hormones need not enter the cell to exert their effects. They work via a variety of second messengers.

Second messengers can be defined as substances which are generated within a cell or which enter its cytosol as a result of the original hormone (first messenger)/receptor interaction, and which then mediate the cellular response. The first of these second

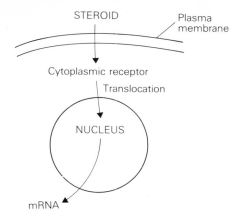

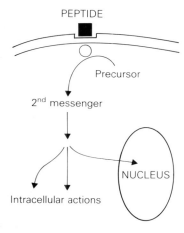

Fig. 1.11 *Mechanism of action of steroid and peptide hormones.*

messengers was discovered in 1958 by Earl Sutherland. In 1965 he proposed the second-messenger hypothesis to explain how adrenaline acts on the liver to increase blood glucose levels (see Chapter 8). The trophic hormone reacts with a specific cell-surface receptor which is linked to the membrane-associated enzyme adenylate cyclase (Fig. 1.12). This is now known to consist of at least two units, an N-protein and a catalytic subunit. The enzyme converts ATP to cyclic AMP which then activates a protein kinase cascade. Cyclic AMP is then degraded to AMP by phosphodiesterase. Thus the cell has a very effective process for

Table 1.2

Hormones Using Cyclic AMP as Second Messenger

Hormone	Target organ	Effect
ACTH	Adrenal	↑ cortisol
LH	Ovary, testis	↑ sex steroids
LHRH	Pituitary	↑ LH and FSH release
TRH	Pituitary	↑ TSH
TSH	Thyroid	↑ T_3, T_4
hCG	Ovary, testis	↑ sex steroids
PTH	Bone	↑ serum calcium
Calcitonin	Bone	↓ serum calcium
Glucagon	Liver	↑ gluconeogenesis
ADH	Kidney	↑ water reabsorption

generating the cAMP necessary for hormone action and for eliminating the second messenger once it has played its role. A wide variety of hormones have now been shown to use cAMP as second messenger (Table 1.2).

However, since the original Sutherland hypothesis was proposed, the picture has become more complicated. Low doses of ACTH, for example, can stimulate steroidogenesis without apparently stimulating cAMP production. These doses, however, increase cyclic GMP by activating guanylate cyclase and it has been proposed that in this situation cGMP acts as the second messenger. One interesting hypothesis to explain this is that there may be two classes of receptor for ACTH which are occupied to different extents depending on the prevailing ACTH concentration, and which are linked to different second messengers. Other hormones thought to stimulate cyclic GMP production are shown in Table 1.3.

Table 1.3

Hormones Using Cyclic GMP as Second Messenger

Hormone	Target organ	Effect
GRF	Pituitary	↑ GH
Adrenaline	Liver	↑ Gluconeogenesis
ACTH	Adrenal cortex	↑ Steroidogenesis

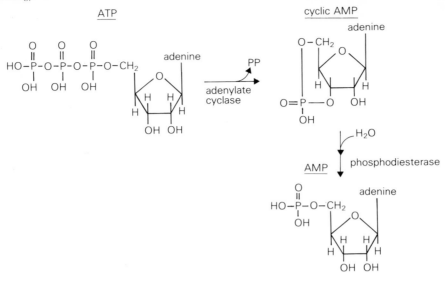

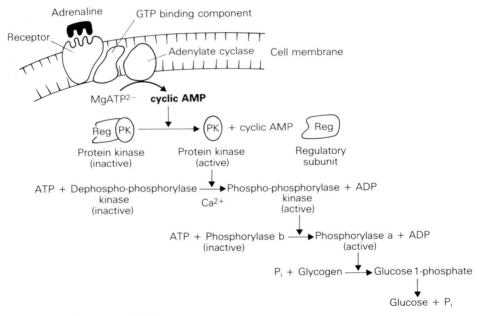

Fig. 1.12 *The conversion of ATP into cyclic AMP by activation of adenylate cyclase and the cascade resulting from stimulation by adrenaline leading to increased glucose production.*

Table 1.4

Hormones Using Calcium as Second Messenger

Hormone	Target organ	Effect
Angiotensin II	Adrenal cortex	↑ aldosterone
Angiotensin II	Smooth muscle	↑ contractility
Adrenaline	Liver	↑ gluconeogenesis
Insulin	Muscle, fat	↑ glucose transport
ACTH	Adrenal cortex	↑ steroidogenesis
Hypothalamic releasing factors	Pituitary	↑ anterior pituitary hormones

critical to understanding the pathophysiology of certain diseases. Parathyroid hormone (PTH), for example, acts by activating adenylate cyclase. One type of hypoparathyroidism is associated with high circulating levels of parathyroid hormone and is hence referred to as pseudohypoparathyroidism. In some of these patients (type I pseudohypoparathyroidism), PTH is unable to activate adenylate cyclase. This can be shown by infusing PTH and demonstrating a failure of the normal rise in urinary cAMP.

After binding to cytoplasmic receptors the lipid soluble hormones (steroids and 1,25-dihydroxyvitamin

The other major second messenger which mediates the action of many hormones is calcium. Table 1.4 lists the hormones using this system. Recent studies using a compound that exhibits a marked increase in fluorescence in the presence of calcium have shown that these hormones produce a rapid increase in intracellular calcium. This can occur by the hormone stimulating a membrane receptor which is linked to a calcium channel (Fig. 1.13). When activated, this allows calcium ions to enter the cell from the extracellular fluid. An alternative possibility is that, when stimulated, the receptor in some way results in calcium release from mitochondria. The increased free ionised calcium activates calcium-dependent enzymes, many of which depend on calmodulin, a calcium receptor present in all mammalian cells.

Figure 1.14 compares the cyclic AMP generating signal which involves a nucleotide regulating protein (N) and adenylate cyclase with the much more complex calcium generating signal. Thus the change in calcium may activate a number of biochemical events including hydrolysis of membrane phospholipids, stimulation of the metabolism of released arachidonic acid to prostaglandins and/or leukotrienes, and the stimulation of guanylate cyclase leading to the increased synthesis of cyclic GMP. The precise involvement of these different mechanisms in various endocrine tissues using calcium as the second messenger is unknown. It has also been shown that changes in calcium transport can be coupled to changes in cyclic AMP via the calcium receptor calmodulin (CaM) which can activate adenylate cyclase in some tissues (Fig. 1.13).

An appreciation of these basic cellular processes is

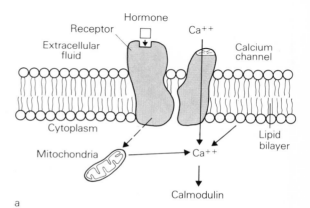

a

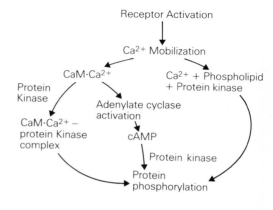

b

Fig. 1.13 *The role of calcium as a second messenger of hormone action.*

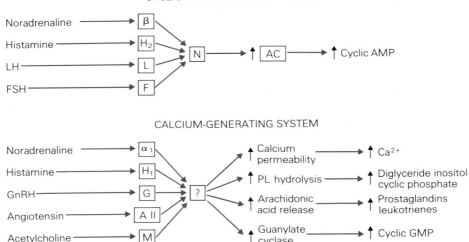

Fig. 1.14 *Comparison of the cyclic AMP-generating system with the calcium-generating system.*

D) are translocated to the nucleus. The receptors are activated when they are bound by the hormone and, in the nucleus, bind to the nuclear acceptors on DNA. This leads to the production of specific messenger RNAs and hence eventually ribosomal protein synthesis. The thyroid hormones differ by not having specific cytoplasmic receptors.

Patterns of Hormone Release

Many hormones are produced in a characteristic pattern and it is important to understand this when investigating and treating endocrine disorders. Adrenocorticotrophin (ACTH) has a marked circadian rhythm, the levels being much higher on waking in the morning as compared to going to bed. This leads to a similar rhythm of cortisol secretion by the adrenals. In Cushing's syndrome, where there is excess production of cortisol by the adrenals, the circadian rhythm is lost (see Chapter 4).

The gonadotrophins luteinising hormone and follicle stimulating hormone are produced in a pulsatile rather than a continuous manner. This is because of the episodic release of the gonadotrophin releasing hormone (GnRH). If long-acting analogues of GnRH are given, this results in so-called 'down regulation' of receptors and hence a loss of pituitary gonadotroph sensitivity. Use can be made of this in treating sex-hormone dependent tumours such as carcinoma of the prostate, and also in contraception. Conversely some patients with infertility such as those with structural or functional hypothalamic disease can be made fertile using a small portable pump which gives injections of GnRH every 90 minutes.

The pattern of hormone release may also be altered by age or weight change. Gonadotrophin secretion in early puberty is principally nocturnal (see Chapter 5). In anorexia nervosa the changes seen during puberty are reversed as weight is lost. A restoration of normal weight will usually be associated with a return of normal gonadotrophin and hence gonadal function.

A variety of factors contribute to the pattern of growth hormone release. Thus a fall in blood sugar will stimulate GH secretion and a rise will suppress it. During sleep large peaks of GH are found related to rapid eye movement. GH secretion may also be increased by 'stress' such as venepuncture. The clinician has to take all these factors into account in assessing the significance of an 'elevated' GH level.

FEEDBACK CONTROL SYSTEMS

Much of the endocrine system can be thought of as a very effective way of amplifying a small signal. For example, the neural input into the hypothalamus stimulates the release of small amounts of a regulatory hormone into the pituitary portal system and hence reaches the anterior pituitary cells (Fig. 1.15). These then secrete larger amounts of a hormone which are then released into the systemic circulation. The target gland then responds to the trophic hormone by producing even greater amounts of its secretory product.

This cascade is in turn modulated by an exquisite system of *negative feedback control*. Thus the product of the pituitary can inhibit the release of the hypothalamic hormone (*short-loop negative feedback*). This compares with the *long-loop negative feedback* when the product of the target gland then controls the secretion of the pituitary and the hypothalamus (see Chapter 2).

Positive-feedback control also exists. The classical example of this is the mid-cycle release of luteinising hormone that triggers ovulation. This is the result of the rising level of oestradiol which stimulates a surge of gonadotrophin releasing hormone and hence LH. The oestrogen however blocks the secretion of follicle stimulating hormone. Thus, even though there is only one gonadotrophin releasing hormone, its interaction with the pituitary and the ovary leads to the different patterns of LH and FSH release that characterise the menstrual cycle (see Chapter 5).

METHODS OF HORMONE MEASUREMENT

Since nearly all modern endocrinology is dependent on accurate measurement of hormone levels it is important for any physician to appreciate something of the methods used. By far the most important of these is radioimmunoassay (Fig. 1.16). This technique depends on the ability of an unlabelled (or 'cold') hormone to displace a fixed amount of radioactively labelled hormone from a limited amount of specific antibody. Thus, in the presence of an excess amount of 'cold' hormone, all the labelled hormone is displaced from the antibody whereas, when there is no 'cold' hormone, there is enough antibody to bind about 50% of the label. Using varying amounts of standard hormone a calibration curve can be constructed and the values of unknown samples read from this curve.

In some assays, binding proteins rather than specific antibodies are used (competitive protein binding assays). In others the labelled compound is not radioactive but fluorescent (fluoroimmunoassay) or linked to an enzyme.

The advantages of radioimmunoassays have been their specificity and sensitivity. It is important, however, to realise that their results do not always equate with those of the more cumbersome bioassays. Thus some tumours which produce ACTH ectopically may secrete C-terminal fragments of the molecule (the species-specific part, Fig. 1.7). If the antibody is directed against an antigenic determinant group in this end of the molecule, it will result in the assay indicating that large amounts of ACTH are being secreted but this will not be biologically active. There is thus a need under certain special circumstances to use bioassays (e.g. the measurement of corticosterone production by a rat adrenal when stimulated by ACTH). The majority of

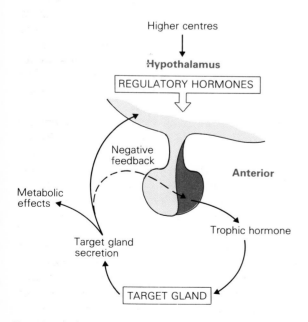

Fig. 1.15 *The hypothalamic–pituitary–target gland axis, indicating negative feedback control by product(s) of the target gland.*

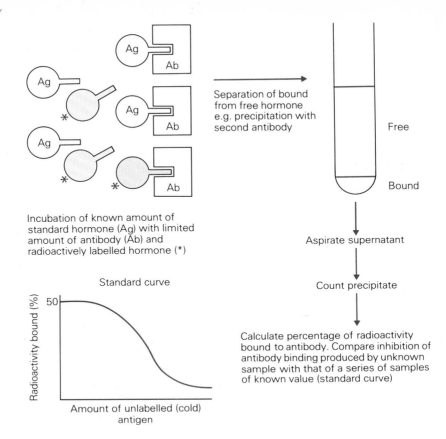

Incubation of known amount of standard hormone (Ag) with limited amount of antibody (Ab) and radioactively labelled hormone (*)

Separation of bound from free hormone e.g. precipitation with second antibody

Free

Bound

Aspirate supernatant

Count precipitate

Calculate percentage of radioactivity bound to antibody. Compare inhibition of antibody binding produced by unknown sample with that of a series of samples of known value (standard curve)

Standard curve

Radioactivity bound (%)

50

Amount of unlabelled (cold) antigen

Fig. 1.16 *The principles of radioimmunoassay.*

these are less sensitive than radioimmunoassays. The exceptions to this are the cytochemical bioassays, many of which are much more sensitive than other assays.

With the advent of the much more specific assay methods such as radioimmunoassay, some of the older ones are being discarded. Thus the techniques used for the so-called group determination of steroids in the urine (17-oxosteroids reflecting androgen secretion and 17-oxogenic steroids as an index of cortisol secretion) are being replaced by assays for the individual androgens and cortisol itself.

Receptor assays depend on the binding of a hormone to its specific receptor. Such binding, however, does not necessarily mean that the substance that binds will produce the normal biological effect of the hormone. If the hormone uses cAMP as its second messenger then measurement of this will suggest that the hormone binding to the receptor is biologically active.

METABOLISM OF HORMONES

Most hormonal systems respond rapidly to the initiating stimulus. A prerequisite of such a system is that the hormone once it has had its effect should be inactivated and excreted. Some hormones (e.g. cortisol) are excreted both as an inactive metabolite such as tetrahydrocortisone and as the active hormone (see Chapter 4). Just as some hormones (e.g. testosterone) are activated by target tissues, these can also serve to inactivate them. The major organ for inactivating hormones is the liver, but some are metabolised by the kidney. After the initial metabolic transformations, hormones such as steroids are frequently then made water-soluble by conjugation with sulphate or glucuronide. They can then be excreted in the bile or urine.

INTRODUCTION TO CLINICAL ENDOCRINOLOGY

Most endocrine diseases can be classified on the basis of being associated either with hormonal excess or hormonal deficiency (Table 1.5). The excess may result from primary overproduction (e.g. by a tumour) or by excessive stimulation of a gland by a trophic substance (e.g. thyroid stimulating antibody producing hyperthyroidism). Hormonal deficiency can arise either from primary failure of the gland or be secondary to a lack of stimulation by a trophic hormone. A rarer cause is where the target organ is resistant to the action of a hormone.

The commonest endocrine diseases are those involving the thyroid gland and that resulting from an absolute or relative lack of insulin (diabetes mellitus). Population screening has shown that many patients have undiagnosed abnormal endocrine function. Many countries now routinely screen all neonates for congenital hypothyroidism (usually by measuring thyroid stimulating hormone on a heel-prick sample). In the United Kingdom the prevalence of this condition is about 1 in 4000 births. This early diagnosis and hence early treatment is critical to minimise the brain damage that is one of the major features of cretinism.

A survey conducted in Whickham, County Durham, was instrumental in showing the spectrum of thyroid disease in a community (see Chapter 3). The survey demonstrated that the prevalence of both hyperthyroidism and hypothyroidism was remarkably high. Overt thyroid overactivity was present in 19/1000 females and in 27/1000 when milder cases were included. This compared with 1.6–2.3/1000 males. Hypothyroidism was found in 14/1000 females and in less than 1/1000 males.

The prevalence of diabetes varies considerably in different parts of the world. In the industrialised nations

Table 1.5

Disorders of the Endocrine System

	Hormonal excess	*Hormonal deficiency*	*Hormonal resistance*
Hypothalamus	?Cushing's disease	Isolated releasing hormone deficiencies for LH, TSH, GH	
Pituitary	Acromegaly Cushing's disease Prolactinoma	Hypopituitarism Diabetes insipidus	Nephrogenic diabetes insipidus Laron dwarfism
Gonad	Tumours	Klinefelter's syndrome Turner's syndrome Menopause	Androgen resistance syndromes (e.g. testicular feminisation)
Thyroid	Hyperthyroidism	Hypothyroidism	Thyroid hormone resistance (very rare)
Adrenal	Cushing's syndrome Conn's syndrome Phaeochromocytoma	Addison's disease	Pseudohypoaldosteronism
Parathyroids	Hyperparathyroidism	Hypoparathyroidism	Pseudohypoparathyroidism
Pancreas	Insulinoma Glucagonoma	Diabetes mellitus	Insulin resistance syndromes

it is approximately 1.5–2% of the population. However, some subgroups such as the North American Indians and the Australian aboriginals have a prevalence in excess of 15% (see Table 8.12, p. 163).

Even though endocrine diseases are a relatively rare cause of death (1–5% according to World Health statistics) they are an important cause of morbidity. This can now largely be prevented. Modern methods of hormone measurement have greatly facilitated the investigation and early diagnosis of endocrine disorders, and the majority of diseases can now be effectively treated. In addition to the classical endocrine conditions there is an increasing awareness of the role that hormones play in many other disease processes. Thus certain cancers, such as those arising in the breast or prostate, may be hormone-dependent (see Chapter 5). Conversely other tumours, such as the small cell carcinoma of the bronchus, may produce hormones ectopically and sometimes present with the endocrine syndrome before the tumour itself becomes manifest (see Chapter 7).

Many endocrine conditions are associated with abnormal functioning of the central nervous system. Patients with Cushing's syndrome, for example, are commonly depressed. Lowering cortisol secretion to normal results in a cure of the depression. In contrast, several psychiatric diseases are associated with abnormal endocrine function. Thus patients with severe depression may have most of the biochemical abnormalities of Cushing's syndrome. At present, however, the role that hormones play in the pathogenesis of psychiatric diseases is unclear. It would seem very likely that they must be important in conditions such as premenstrual tension and post-partum depression.

The field of neuroendocrinology is one of the most rapidly growing areas of endocrinology. The isolation and synthesis of the regulatory hormones of the hypothalamus has had an immediate impact on clinical practice (see Chapter 2). The discovery that the brain has its own endogenous opiate system (the endorphins and the enkephalins) has been a major stimulus to workers in this area. We are only beginning to understand that these brain hormones may have several roles. Thus opiates appear to be important not only in the body's reaction to pain but also, for example, in controlling the pulsatile release of gonadotrophin releasing hormone. Other work has suggested that the antidiuretic hormone, arginine vasopressin, may play an integral part in learning and memory in addition to its action on the kidney. The way in which hormones have adapted to perform a variety of functions in different parts of the body is one of the fascinations of endocrinology.

2

The Hypothalamus, Anterior and Posterior Pituitary

INTRODUCTION

In the past decade, rapid advances have occurred in our knowledge of the hypothalamus and pituitary. Precise measurement of circulating hormones has become possible through radioimmunoassay (RIA), thus enabling accurate assessment of function and treatment to occur. More recently, prolactin has been discovered to exist as a separate hormone in man, and a whole range of clinical problems are now known to be associated with hyperprolactinaemia, which is common. Furthermore, a number of hypothalamic hormones have been isolated, characterised and synthesised, thus increasing our knowledge of the mechanisms whereby the hypothalamus controls the pituitary and also giving us tools in the diagnosis and treatment of disease in this area.

This chapter will discuss the causes, diagnosis and treatment of pituitary diseases in the light of these exciting and significant advances. The first half of the chapter will deal with the foundations of the subject in terms of anatomy and physiology, and the second will integrate these and show how physiological advances have been applied to clinical practice.

ANATOMY AND PHYSIOLOGY OF THE HYPOTHALAMUS AND PITUITARY

Anatomy

The pituitary gland consists of anterior and posterior lobes, which have a separate origin and function independently. The anterior lobe (adenohypophysis) develops from an ectodermal evagination of the oropharynx (Rathke's pouch). This grows up from the stomadeal roof and becomes separated from it to form a vesicle from which the adenohypophysis is formed. The posterior lobe develops from a downgrowth of the diencephalic portion of the forebrain (the infundibulum). This meets Rathke's pouch and forms the neurohypophysis. The upper part of Rathke's pouch forms the pars tuberalis of the anterior pituitary gland that partly encircles the pituitary stalk (Fig. 2.1). This structure is well-developed in man, compared with other animals, and explains the occasional development of pituitary tumours above the diaphragma sellae. The posterior part of Rathke's pouch forms the

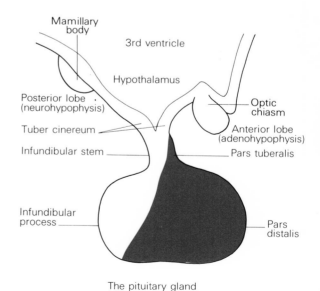

The pituitary gland

Fig. 2.1 *The anatomy of the hypothalamus and pituitary gland.*

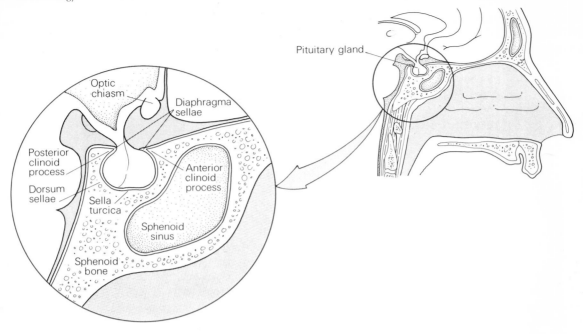

Fig. 2.2 *The relationship of the pituitary gland to surrounding structures.*

pars intermedia in lower animals, but this is rudimentary in man. The anterior part forms the pars distalis. The neurohypophysis consists of three parts: the median eminence or tuber cinereum which goes back as far as the mamillary bodies; the infundibular stem; and the infundibular process. The posterior pituitary contains nerve fibres which grow into it via the stalk from the hypothalamic nuclei in the base and lateral walls of the third ventricle.

The main body of the pituitary gland lies in a deep recess of the sphenoid bone, called the sella turcica or pituitary fossa, the posterior wall of which is named the dorsum sellae (Fig. 2.2). The pituitary is connected to the hypothalamus by the stalk, which carries axons to the neurohypophysis and blood vessels to both parts. Laterally the gland is bounded by the cavernous sinus, on the lateral wall of which are the IIIrd, IVth and VIth cranial nerves and the carotid syphon. It is roofed by dura mater, which forms the diaphragma sellae; this contains an opening for the pituitary stalk. Above the diaphragma lie the optic nerves, chiasm and tracts, and

above this the hypothalamus and the third ventricle. Beneath the pituitary lies the sphenoid air sinus.

The gland weighs between 0·5 and 0·9 g. It is larger in the female, especially in parous women because oestrogen stimulates the prolactin-producing cells (lactotrophs), and smaller in old age. The pars distalis, which forms about three-quarters of the pituitary, consists of cuboidal epithelial cells through which traverse a profuse network of sinusoids. These cells vary in size, in staining characteristics, and in content of the intracellular granules containing hormone (Table 2.1). The original haematoxylin and eosin (H and E) stains that indicated acidophil (red-staining granules), basophil (purple-staining granules), and chromophobe (non-staining) regions of the cell were superseded in the 1950s by more complex stains, and histochemical methods, which rely on less subjective criteria than apparent colour. Electron microscopy demonstrated granules of differing average sizes containing hormones in these cells. Finally, immunofluorescence methods became available, in which antibodies to the various

Table 2.1

Staining Characteristics and Granule Size of the Anterior Pituitary

	H & E	PAS-OG	Mean granule diameter (nm)
1. Growth hormone (GH)	acidophil	yellow	450
2. Prolactin	acidophil	yellow	550
3. Thyroid stimulating hormone (TSH)	basophil	magenta	135
4. Luteinising hormone (LH) Follicle stimulating hormone (FSH)	basophil	magenta	200
5. Adrenocorticotrophic hormone (ACTH) β-lipotrophin (LPH)	basophil	magenta	360

pituitary hormones are attached to fluorescent dyes that can be seen under the microscope.

This technique of immunostaining has now been used to identify five separate cell types, containing the following hormones: growth hormone (GH); prolactin (Prl); thyrotrophic hormone (TSH); the gonadotrophic hormones follicle stimulating hormone (FSH) and luteinising hormone (LH); and finally adrenocorticotrophic hormone (ACTH) plus β-lipotrophin (β-LPH).

The most useful modern routine histological staining technique is the periodic acid–Schiff–orange G (PAS–OG) stain. This stains acidophils yellow and basophils various intensities of magenta. PAS-positive

cells have been named mucoid cells, reflecting the glycoprotein nature of their granules, which fits the glycoprotein composition of TSH, FSH and LH. Examination of normal anterior pituitary in the electron microscope shows that all, or practically all, the cells contain secretory granules. Examination by light microscopy shows that the number of chromophobic cells is small or zero. Sparsely granulated chromophobe cells are either very actively secreting or else resting.

The infundibular process of the posterior pituitary gland is the terminal expansion of the neural component of the pituitary. It contains blood vessels, pituicytes resembling neuroglial cells elsewhere in the

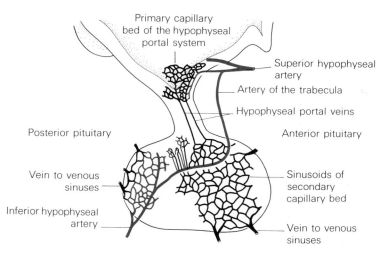

Fig. 2.3 *The blood supply of the pituitary gland.*

nervous system and nerve fibres mainly from the supraoptic and paraventricular nuclei of the hypothalamus. The cells of these nuclei in the hypothalamus are neurosecretory and produce oxytocin and vasopressin. These hormones pass down the nerve fibres and can be seen as stainable neurosecretory material in the posterior pituitary, from whence they are released.

The blood supply of the pituitary comes from two main sources above and below the diaphragma sellae (Fig. 2.3). These are the superior and inferior hypophyseal arteries, which are both paired and arise from the internal carotid artery. Characteristic vascular arrangements are found in each part of the pituitary. In the median eminence and upper pituitary stalk, there are coiled capillary loops fed by branches of the superior hypophyseal artery (primary capillaries). These do not drain into the general circulation but form a portal system through long straight venous vessels which run down the stalk into the pars distalis and from there into the sinusoids of that lobe. These are the long portal vessels of the hypophyseal portal system and provide the pars distalis, the largest part of the anterior pituitary, with the majority of its exclusively portal blood supply. It is now accepted that hypothalamic secretions from nerve endings near the primary capillary bed pass from these into the portal capillaries from where they stimulate or inhibit the parenchymal cells of the pars distalis. Blood drains from the sinusoids into the local surrounding venous sinuses. The capillary network in the infundibular process of the posterior pituitary is supplied by the inferior hypophyseal artery in a conventional manner and there is no portal circulation. These capillaries are much smaller than the sinusoids of the pars distalis.

THE HYPOTHALAMIC CONTROL OF PITUITARY FUNCTION

This is one of the areas of endocrinology where major discoveries in the last few years, particularly the characterisation of some of the hypothalamic hormones, have had profound implications for our understanding of the physiology of hypothalamic and pituitary function.

It was known at the end of the last century that the infundibular process of the posterior pituitary contained a substance which, when injected into animals, produced a rise in blood pressure, and which was called vasopressin. Soon after, it was discovered that the posterior pituitary contained another substance which could stimulate uterine contraction. This was given the name of oxytocin. The pars distalis was also known to contain hormones but the control and the means of their production and release were obscure. The work of Geoffrey Harris in Oxford in the second quarter of this century laid the foundations of our present knowledge of the hypothalamic control of anterior pituitary function. The neuroendocrine role of the hypothalamus was initially studied by observing the effects of ablation and electrical stimulation. Thus lesions of the hypothalamus could be shown to disrupt the menstrual cycle and electrical stimulation could evoke ovulation in one area, and thyroid hormone secretion in another. Experiments of this nature have been used to localise the function of different areas of the hypothalamus.

It is now known that the major role of the hypothalamus is to act as an integrating centre between the higher centres of the brain and the pituitary. Besides regulating pituitary function, the hypothalamus controls sexual activity, body temperature, appetite and water balance. It lies below the thalamus (Fig. 2.4) and, although its limits are poorly defined, the major part is in the tissues surrounding the lower part of the third ventricle. Much of the anatomy of the hypothalamic neural connections is known but little is understood of their function. Thus, extracts of sheep, bovine and pig hypothalamus have been shown to contain factors (or hormones) that can influence the release of anterior pituitary hormones both *in vivo* and *in vitro*. They can also be measured in blood removed from the portal circulation. It seems clear that the hypothalamus controls the anterior pituitary by the release of these small molecules into the portal circulation. The release of these hormones is in turn controlled by nerve terminals close to the capillaries where they are released. The terminals contain a number of neurotransmitters, e.g. noradrenaline, dopamine, acetylcholine, gamma-aminobutyric acid, and enkephalin. There are no neural connections between the hypothalamus and anterior pituitary, and the only control appears to be humoral. Anterior pituitary hormones released as a result of these stimuli can stimulate the target organ and hormone release from this can, by negative feedback probably at both the pituitary and hypothala-

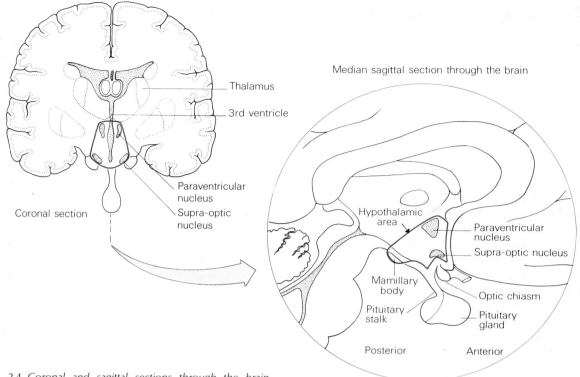

Fig. 2.4 *Coronal and sagittal sections through the brain, showing the anatomy of the hypothalamus.*

mic levels, switch off hypothalamic and anterior pituitary hormone production.

THE HYPOTHALAMIC HORMONES

Thyrotrophin Releasing Hormone (TRH)

This, in 1969, was the first hypothalamic hormone to be isolated. It is a tripeptide which, when given intravenously, causes the secretion of both TSH and prolactin. It is clearly of importance in the regulation of TSH secretion but its physiological significance in the control of prolactin secretion is as yet unclear. The main clinical use of this hormone is in the diagnosis of thyroid disease. Normally, after the administration of

200 μg TRH intravenously, there is a peak of TSH at 20 minutes and then a subsequent fall at 60 minutes (Fig. 2.6). In hyperthyroid patients, however, there is no increase in TSH. This is because of autonomous thyroid function, e.g. in Graves' disease as a result of stimulation with thyroid stimulating antibodies, or in the presence of an autonomously functioning adenoma. The elevated levels of thyroid hormone suppress the hypothalamus and pituitary and hence, when TRH is given, no rise in TSH is seen. Other causes of a flat TSH response to TRH (besides autonomous thyroid hyperfunction) include patients on T_4 therapy, those with euthyroid ophthalmic Graves' disease, euthyroid multinodular goitre, hypopituitarism, and patients on high-dose corticosteroid therapy.

In hypothyroidism due to primary thyroid disease, there is an exaggerated rise in TSH after TRH. In

RELEASING   INHIBITING

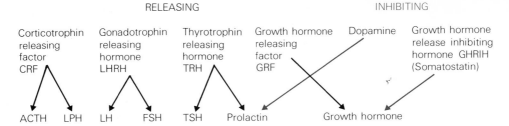

Fig. 2.5 *The releasing and inhibiting hormones and factors of the hypothalamus.*

hypothyroidism with pituitary or hypothalamic disease (secondary hypothyroidism), the TRH test is less useful since a rise in TSH may still be seen in the presence of a low circulating thyroxine concentration. Lastly, TRH has been used to assess prolactin reserve. However, states of prolactin deficiency are not clinically important: hyperprolactinaemia is much commoner. When this is due to a prolactin-secreting pituitary tumour, the prolactin response to TRH may be impaired, but the diagnosis of a prolactinoma is probably best made on the basis of the unstimulated level of serum prolactin.

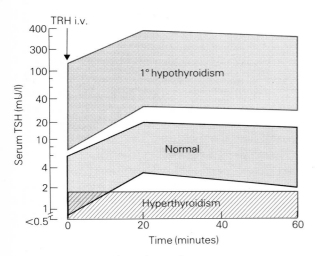

Fig. 2.6 *The thyrotrophin releasing hormone test.*

Gonadotrophin Releasing Hormone (GnRH, LHRH)

This was the second hypothalamic hormone to be isolated. It is a decapeptide and causes the release of both LH and FSH. LHRH is also responsible for the synthesis of LH and FSH in the basophil cells of the anterior pituitary. It is essential for complete pubertal development, which does not take place if there is deficiency of LHRH (Kallman's syndrome).

At different stages in puberty, the pituitary gonadotrophs show varying responses to intravenous LHRH (GnRH). In the early stages there is a greater rise in FSH than LH but, as puberty progresses, this changes so that in later puberty the LH rise is greater than that of FSH.

LHRH may help in the diagnosis of pituitary disease. Clearly, basal levels of gonadotrophin are sufficient for some diagnoses, e.g. primary gonadal failure when the LH and FSH levels are both very high. In pituitary disease, however, intravenous administration of LHRH may help in the diagnosis of LH deficiency. This is particularly important because, in progressive pituitary failure, LH secretion is frequently the first of the trophic hormones to become deficient.

Somatostatin (Growth Hormone Release Inhibiting Hormone, GHRIH)

This tetradecapeptide is present in highest concentrations in the hypothalamus, where it acts as a true hormone, and is also found in other areas of the brain where it may act as a neurotransmitter. It inhibits growth hormone by direct action on the pituitary. Presumably growth hormone control is brought about by interaction of somatostatin and growth hormone releasing factor (GRF), which has very recently been characterised. GRF appears to be the predominant of these two hormones. Somatostatin is widely distributed both in the central and peripheral nervous systems and the gut. In the latter it is present in high concentrations in the pyloric antrum and pancreatic D cells where it may act as a paracrine hormone (i.e. it controls other cells by means of intercellular diffusion rather than by the more classical endocrine means). By this process somatostatin regulates insulin and glucagon secretion from the pancreatic islet.

When administered intravenously, somatostatin inhibits the secretion of a large number of gastrointestinal hormones and secretions including insulin, glucagon and gastrin. The physiological significance of these actions is unclear, because the doses that have been administered result in very high supraphysiological levels of somatostatin in the circulation.

Growth Hormone Releasing Factor (GRF)

Two growth hormone releasing factors have recently been identified in two pancreatic tumours secreting this hormone and causing acromegaly. One tumour produced a 40-amino-acid linear peptide and the other a 44-amino-acid molecule. The first 40 amino acids are common to both. The molecules have now been synthesised. The GRF 1–40 releases growth hormone in animals and man. It also stimulates GH release in subjects with isolated growth hormone deficiency suggesting that this disorder is probably a hypothalamic disease. This raises the possibility that children with GH deficiency could be treated with GRF.

Corticotrophin Releasing Factor (CRF)

This hormone, a 41-amino-acid peptide, was isolated in 1981. It stimulates the secretion of only ACTH and β-lipotrophin. It is probable that this is not the only corticotrophin releasing factor, and there is some evidence that vasopressin is also important in the release of ACTH and β-LPH from the anterior pituitary.

The clinical significance and uses of this peptide are currently being evaluated in man.

Prolactin Inhibiting Factor

Prolactin is under the inhibitory control of the hypothalamus. It is the only hormone in the anterior pituitary to be controlled in this way: thus stalk section results in hyperprolactinaemia but a fall in the circulating levels of all the other anterior pituitary trophic hormones. It is probable that the prolactin inhibiting factor is dopamine. Certainly dopamine in concentrations that are present in the hypophyseal portal circulation inhibits prolactin secretion *in vitro,* and there are known to be dopamine receptors on the anterior pituitary. This explains why drugs which act on dopamine receptors (e.g. bromocriptine) alter prolactin secretion.

ANTERIOR PITUITARY HORMONES

Prolactin (Table 2.2)

Prolactin, the hormone responsible for the unique mammalian trait of lactation, was first discovered to exist as a separate entity in man in 1970. It acts on the prepared breast to stimulate growth and support the secretion of milk. Hypersecretion of this hormone is a common clinical problem resulting in a wide range of disorders in both men and women.

The main understood effect of prolactin is to initiate lactation. Thus the most profound changes in the serum concentration of prolactin occur during pregnancy and lactation and the concentration of prolactin increases progressively up to tenfold through pregnancy and remains elevated during lactation. Nipple stimulation acts via a neural reflex arc to cause a rise in prolactin. Any form of nipple stimulus may do this and it does not occur if, as has been shown in goats, the nipple is denervated. Normal lactation also requires the presence of adequate amounts of thyroxine, oestradiol, progesterone and oxytocin. A number of other actions are known in other species, where prolactin may be somatotrophic, have effects on salt and water balance, and affect behaviour. The exact significance of these actions in man is, however, at present uncertain.

Table 2.2

The Anterior Pituitary Hormones

Hormone	Site of action	Action
Prolactin	Breast	Lactation
GH	1. Liver	Somatomedin production, growth
	2. Metabolic effects	Protein synthesis, anti-insulin effect
ACTH	1. Adrenal cortex	Cortisol production
		Maintenance of adrenal weight
	2. Skin	?Pigmentation
LPH	?	?precursor of β-endorphin ?pigmentation
TSH	Thyroid follicle	Thyroxine (T_4) production
		Tri-iodothyronine (T_3) production
LH	1. Ovarian follicle	Ovulation, corpus luteum and progesterone production
	2. Interstitial cells	Testosterone production
FSH	1. Ovarian follicle	Oestrogen production
	2. Seminiferous tubules	Spermatogenesis

Prolactin is a single-chain polypeptide hormone chemically related to growth hormone. It is for this reason that it was difficult to differentiate the two in man. It circulates and can now be reliably measured by radioimmunoassay. Although values from different laboratories may vary, values above 400 mU/l (20 ng/ml) are probably abnormal. Values tend to be higher in women than in men because oestrogen stimulates anterior pituitary prolactin secretion. There is a circadian rhythm and highest values are seen at night. Superimposed on this, its secretion is pulsatile. Of great importance is the fact that this hormone is a stress hormone. Therefore, when assessing prolactin secretion, it is important that fear and pain are obviated during venesection since the presence of either of these two factors will elevate the circulating level.

Growth Hormone (GH) Somatotrophic Hormone

This is a single-chain peptide that has two intrachain disulphide bridges and consists of 191 amino acids. It is species specific so that the administration of bovine growth hormone to man does not cause human growth because of a difference of several amino acids. It is one of the major products of the human pituitary, from which 5–10 mg of growth hormone can be extracted. As a result of earlier radioimmunoassay work, we now know a great deal about the physiology and control of growth hormone secretion. Except in the newborn, levels are low (< 2 mU/l (1 ng/ml)) during the day. It is secreted in bursts which last from minutes to several hours. The half-life in the circulation is around 25 minutes. Major growth hormone secretion occurs at night during EEG stages 3 and 4 of sleep (deep sleep), and these bursts are higher in growing children and during adolescence. Despite the paroxysms of secretion, the effects of GH are smoothed out by the fact that GH, which can influence a variety of tissues, stimulates the production of somatomedins, a group of large-molecular-weight peptides (6000–8000 daltons) produced mainly in the liver, which are directly responsible for growth. It is also a stress hormone and circulating levels rise in response to exercise. Another major cause of secretion is a fall in blood sugar. Conversely, there is a fall in GH secretion after a glucose load. Some amino acids also cause a rise in growth hormone, the most notable of these being arginine. Pharmacological doses of corticosteroids cause a decrease in growth hormone secretion, and this may be one of the reasons why children on supraphysiological doses of these drugs do not grow normally. A number of neurotransmitters are important in the modulation of growth hormone and these include noradrenaline, dopamine and serotonin. Thus drugs which effect these neurotransmitters effect growth hormone levels either basally or in response to various stimuli. For example, dopamine receptor agonists in normal subjects transiently raise serum growth hormone.

Adrenocorticotrophic Hormone (ACTH)

This is a single-chain polypeptide consisting of 39 amino acids; it has a molecular weight of 4500. The N-terminal 24 amino acids are required for stimulating the adrenal cortex; amino acids 25–39 are responsible for species specificity. ACTH is one of a family of related peptides that are derived from a larger precursor glycoprotein, of molecular weight 31 000, called pro-opiocortin. Other derivatives are the melanocyte stimulating hormones (MSH), lipotrophin molecules, enkephalins and endorphins (Fig. 2.7).

Besides steroidogenesis, ACTH can cause skin pigmentation such as that seen in Addison's disease, and when there is ectopic ACTH production by malignant tumours. It is probable that ACTH is not responsible for the maintenance of adrenal weight. This may be a function of the N-terminal part of pro-opiocortin. Some animal species secrete α-MSH (melanocyte stimulating hormone) from the anterior pituitary gland. This hormone is chemically related to ACTH (Fig. 2.7). It does not circulate in man and is not, as was previously supposed, responsible for skin pigmentation in man.

Lipotrophins

The secretion of ACTH is under the hypothalamic control of corticotrophin releasing factor (CRF). ACTH exhibits a circadian rhythm, with a nadir at midnight and a peak of secretion between 0600 and 0800 hours. This is disturbed in Cushing's syndrome, heart failure, depression, stress and any serious illness. Besides its circadian rhythm, ACTH levels are dependent, via a negative feedback system, on levels of circulating cortisol. The third important factor modulating secretion is stress (including hypoglycaemic stress) which overrides both the circadian rhythm and the feedback control. By radioimmunoassay, levels of ACTH in normal subjects vary between 10–80 ng/l at 0900 and become undetectable (< 10 ng/l) at midnight. Measurements of this hormone are of importance in the differential diagnosis of Cushing's syndrome and in the diagnosis of Addison's disease. Because it is unstable in plasma, plasma samples for ACTH measurement must be frozen as soon as possible after venepuncture.

There are two lipotrophins, beta and gamma lipotrophin (Fig. 2.7). These originate from the same cells as ACTH but have little pigmentary activity. Beta LPH has 91 amino acids, and gamma LPH has the first 58 of these. The name lipotrophin was given because it was initially thought that the hormone had fat mobilising activities. Its true function, however, is at present unknown, but it is of great interest that its sequence contains the endogenous peptides which in man relieve pain, particularly the endorphins (*endo*genous *morphin*e) and met-enkephalin.

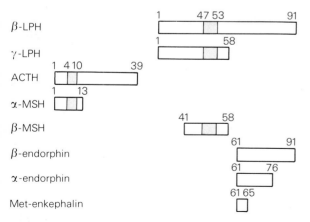

Fig. 2.7 *Peptides derived from the ACTH precursor molecule pro-opiocortin. The shaded area indicates a common MSH sequence. Even though the met-enkephalin sequence is contained within β-LPH, β-endorphin and α-endorphin it is not thought to be derived from these peptides.*

Thyroid Stimulating Hormone (TSH)

This is a glycoprotein hormone (containing both carbohydrate and protein) which, like LH, FSH and human chorionic gonadotrophin (HCG, from the placenta), has separate α and β subunits. It has a molecular weight of about 28 000. The α subunits of these four hormones are effectively identical but the β subunits – which are not alike – are responsible for their biological and immunological specificities.

TSH is under the stimulatory control of TRH, and feedback is under the inhibitory control of the thyroid hormones, predominantly tri-iodothyronine (T_3). TSH secretion has a circadian rhythm; levels rise about 2 hours after sleep to peak between 0200 and 0400 hours. Superimposed upon this are oscillations caused by episodic secretion.

TSH stimulates secretion of tri-iodothyronine (T_3) and thyroxine (T_4). It also stimulates almost all of the metabolic processes in the thyroid gland, including iodide trapping and the formation and the release of the thyroid hormones. TSH can be measured by radioimmunoassay and these measurements are of great value in clinical practice. TSH secretion is low in hyperthyroidism. The recent introduction of much more sensitive TSH assays has enabled the distinction of subnormal from normal TSH values. Prior to the introduction of these the demonstration of thyroid autonomy depended on the TRH test. TSH levels are high in primary hypothyroidism. In hypothyroidism due to pituitary failure, on the other hand, TSH levels are not elevated, but are normal or low. Serum TSH levels are also used to assess the adequacy of thyroxine replacement in primary hypothyroidism, when the pituitary thyrotroph will stop producing TSH as soon as adequate thyroxine is being taken.

Gonadotrophins

The gonadotrophins, like TSH, are glycoprotein hormones, containing both an α and β chain, and are secreted by the same cell of the pituitary. Luteinising hormone (LH) in females induces ovulation, stimulates oestrogen and progesterone production from the ovary, and initiates and maintains the corpus luteum. In males it stimulates the interstitial Leydig cells of the testis to produce androgens. Human chorionic gonadotrophin (HCG) is structurally closely related to LH and is produced by the human placenta and some ovarian and testicular tumours of trophoblastic origin. It has a predominantly luteinising action, and its presence can be used as an early specific pregnancy test. Follicle stimulating hormone (FSH) stimulates the ovarian primordial follicle. It also stimulates the ovary's granulosa cells to proliferate. In the male, FSH stimulates seminiferous tubule development and spermatogenesis, through the mediation of the Sertoli cells of the testis.

In infancy, levels of both FSH and LH are low, but those of FSH are greater than LH. As puberty begins, FSH levels rise; in the next stages of puberty the LH levels rise so that, by the end of puberty, they are higher than those of FSH. Initially there are peaks of LH at night but these eventually occur intermittently throughout the whole 24 hours. In the adult, levels of both hormones (but particularly LH) are pulsatile although they show no circadian rhythm. In adult women, there is a well-recognised cyclical variation of LH and FSH secretion. Both hormones are very high postmenopausally but LH continues to be secreted in a pulsatile manner at a rate of one to two pulses per hour. The feedback control of gonadotrophin production is complex and inadequately documented in males. In premenopausal women there are both negative and positive effects of gonadal steroids on gonadotrophin secretion. In the follicular and luteal phases of the cycle (Fig. 2.8), basal gonadotrophin secretion is controlled by a classical negative feedback action of oestradiol. Immature follicles respond in the follicular phase to the gonadotrophin stimulus by increasing in size and secreting increasing quantities of oestradiol, which is maximal near to midcycle. When oestradiol exceeds a certain threshold for a prolonged time (36 hours), the negative feedback action of the steroid is interrupted and oestradiol now causes the discharge of the preovulatory gonadotrophin surge, which is a positive feedback effect. After this, normal gonadotrophin secretion is resumed. In males, on the other hand, there is negative feedback only. It is also suggested that there is a further substance, inhibin, which is important in the feedback inhibition of FSH. This substance, which is as yet uncharacterised in man, is probably produced by the seminiferous tubules and secreted as the sperms mature. FSH levels are high therefore in azoospermia.

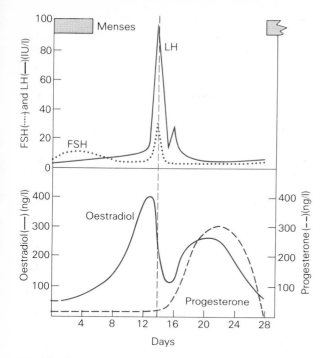

Fig. 2.8 *The secretory pattern of gonadotrophins and sex steroids during the normal female menstrual cycle.*

Gonadotrophin assays are of use in the differentiation of pituitary and hypothalamic versus gonadal disease in patients with hypogonadism. They are also of assistance in assessing the stage of pubertal development.

POSTERIOR PITUITARY HORMONES

Vasopressin and oxytocin are synthesised in the supraoptic and paraventricular nuclei of the hypothalamus. These neurosecretions are transported down the stalk together with transport proteins, the neurophysins, and are stored in the neurohypophysis in secretory terminals and released directly into the blood stream. These hormones circulate unbound in the blood and so are removed rapidly from the circulation, mainly by the kidney. They have a half-life of about 5 minutes. Vasopressin (antidiuretic hormone, ADH) is a cyclic peptide of 9 amino acids, molecular weight about 1000, and differs by only two amino acids from oxytocin, thus explaining the similarity of actions of these two pituitary hormones. The action of vasopressin (ADH) is to promote renal tubular reabsorption of water by increasing the permeability of the cells lining the distal tubule and collecting ducts. The renal tubules may be genetically unresponsive to the hormone (nephrogenic diabetes insipidus). Hypokalaemia, hypercalcaemia and amyloidosis also render the renal tubules unresponsive to ADH, thus explaining why polyuria may occur in these conditions. The actions of ADH on the distal tubule are inhibited by lithium and demethylchlortetracycline (these drugs can cause polyuria), and potentiated by chlorpropramide which may help in the treatment of partial ADH deficiency. Vasopressin has the additional action of stimulating smooth muscle contraction and, in pharmacological doses, causes pallor, coronary constriction and contraction of the smooth muscle in the gut.

Release of vasopressin is caused by a rise in osmolality and this is the major factor involved in its control. The osmolality is quite tightly controlled between 280 and 288 mosmol/kg through osmoreceptors in the hypothalamus. Other factors stimulate the secretion of vasopressin, including a fall in blood volume and hypotension (probably because of baroreceptors in the carotid sinus, aortic area and left atrium), emotional factors, stress, pain, trauma (e.g. during surgery) and exercise. Nicotine and morphine stimulate vasopressin release, and alcohol has an antidiuretic effect.

Oxytocin cannot normally be detected in the circulation but levels are episodically elevated during parturition, lactation and coitus. Vaginal distension causes oxytocin release, as does the nipple stimulation during suckling which leads to ejection of milk. Oxytocin thus has actions which are mainly confined to the uterus and breast in animals. The control of secretion in man is currently uncertain partly because it is difficult to measure circulating concentrations. At present there are no recognised syndromes associated with increased or decreased oxytocin secretion.

PITUITARY TUMOURS

Pituitary tumours are almost always benign and may arise from elements of the anterior or posterior pituitary or from the remnants of the craniopharyngeal pouch. Parapituitary tumours (i.e. in the region around the pituitary) also occur, but together with infiltrations and granulomas in this region, are much less common (Table 2.3). Some of the infiltrations and infections listed may not only involve parapituitary structures, such as the hypothalamus, but also the pituitary itself.

Small pituitary tumours (microadenomas) are present in one-quarter of all patients examined at autopsy, but the functional significance of these is at present unknown. Pituitary tumours account for 10% of clinically significant intracranial neoplasms.

Anterior pituitary tumours are benign epithelial tumours and consist of chromophobe, acidophil and basophil adenomas (based on the staining characteristics already mentioned). Chromophobe adenomas are the commonest and are usually the largest of the pituitary tumours that are seen. They have an equal sex incidence and are rare in childhood. They may be part of a multiple endocrine adenoma syndrome (MEA) and associated with other endocrine adenomas, e.g. parathyroid or pancreatic adenomas. Some of these tumours secrete no hormone and are called functionless. Seventy per cent of chromophobe adenomas are associated with hyperprolactinaemia, though in some this is mild (< 1000 mU/l) and probably associated with pressure of the tumour on the pituitary stalk and portal circulation, which interferes with the inhibitory control of the hypothalamus on the pituitary. Growth hormone and ACTH may also be secreted independently by these adenomas. They may also secrete more than one hormone simultaneously, e.g. growth hormone and prolactin.

Acidophil adenomas are smaller and are usually associated with acromegaly or hyperprolactinaemia. Basophil adenomas occur with the least frequency and are the smallest of tumours that occur in the pituitary; they rarely produce pituitary expansion radiologically and are usually associated with Cushing's disease. Tumours secreting the glycoprotein hormones, TSH, LH and FSH, occur but are very rare, as are posterior pituitary tumours. Craniopharyngiomas (tumours arising from the remnants of Rathke's pouch) are not uncommon, classically occurring in children and adolescents; the majority show calcification above the sella

---

Table 2.3

Pituitary and Parapituitary Lesions

Pituitary	Parapituitary
Anterior pituitary	Pinealoma (ectopic)
Functioning	Secondary deposits; breast, lung
Prolactin secreting	Reticulosis
Growth hormone secreting	Optic nerve glioma
ACTH secreting	Sphenoidal ridge meningioma
TSH or gonadotrophin secreting	
– very rare	
Non-functioning	Infiltrations
Chromophobe adenoma	Sarcoidosis
Sarcoma	Histiocytosis
Posterior pituitary	Haemochromatosis
Craniopharyngioma	
Astrocytoma – very rare	Infections
Ganglioneuroma	Tuberculosis
	Abscess
	Syphilis

turcica on plain skull x-ray. These tumours may be cystic or solid and histologically are lined with squamous epithelium.

Clinical Manifestations

Local pressure

Headaches are frequent with pituitary tumours, but vary in their location and severity. They may be due to stretching of the dura above the pituitary or, in the presence of hypothalamic lesions, to the development of hydrocephalus. Visual disturbances are the most typical abnormality, usually due to a suprasellar extension of the tumour (Fig. 2.9). Usually, upper temporal field defects occur first but the exact abnormality depends upon the position of the optic chiasm in relation to the tumour and on the exact part of the pituitary that enlarges. A decrease in visual acuity may occur and it is therefore essential to test the fields of all patients with decreased visual acuity as this may be the presenting feature of a pituitary tumour. With long-standing pressure on the chiasm, optic atrophy and blindness occur which are usually irreversible. Hypothalamic involvement may cause diabetes insipidus, and this is most frequently seen with craniopharyngiomas. Obesity and sleep disturbances may occur but are less common symptoms of hypothalamic

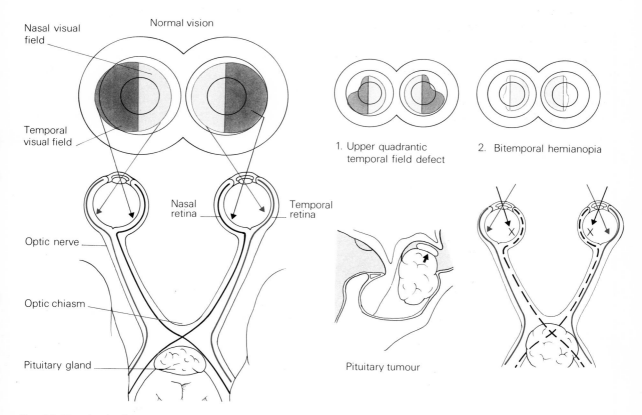

Fig. 2.9 *The local effects of a pituitary tumour; a small suprasellar extension pressing on the inferior fibres crossing in the optic chiasm will produce an upper quadrantic field defect. Further enlargement of the tumour will lead to a bitemporal hemianopia.*

Lateral extension causing –

Cranial nerve palsies   Temporal lobe epilepsy

(a)

Oculomotor
nerve III

Trochlear
nerve IV

Abducens
nerve VI

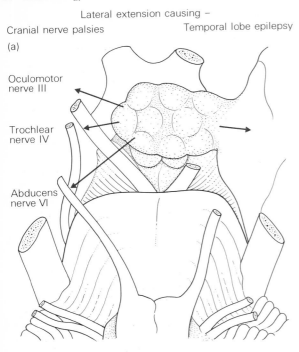

Downward extension causing
cerebrospinal fluid rhinorrhoea

(b)

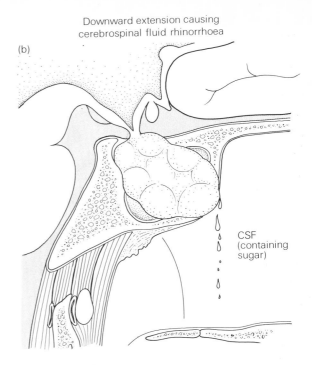

CSF
(containing
sugar)

Fig. 2.10 *Lateral extension of a pituitary tumour into the cavernous sinus may produce cranial nerve palsies. Occasional tumours will further extend, and present with temporal lobe epilepsy. Erosion of the floor may cause a nasal leak of cerebrospinal fluid (CSF).*

disturbance. Lateral extension of the tumour into the cavernous sinus causes interference in the function of the IIIrd, and sometimes the IVth and VIth cranial nerves (Fig. 2.10). Big extensions may cause temporal lobe epilepsy but this is very rare indeed. CSF rhinorrhoea due to inferior extension of the tumour is very rare, but pituitary tumours may erode the sphenoid bone and appear in the sphenoid sinus or post-nasal space.

Hormonal changes

These also occur with great frequency in patients with pituitary tumours. As stated above pituitary tumours may be functionless, and produce deficiencies of the anterior and, very occasionally, posterior pituitary hormones (hypopituitarism) due to compression of the surrounding pituitary. If the pituitary tumour is functioning, there may be a mixed picture due to the effects of the oversecreted hormone plus or minus those of hypopituitarism. All cases therefore need detailed endocrinological evaluation to determine whether there is hormone excess or deficiency.

HYPOPITUITARISM

Hypopituitarism is most commonly caused by a pituitary tumour, but there are other causes. Thus, all pituitary and parapituitary tumours and lesions listed in Table 2.3 may be associated with hypopituitarism. In addition, massive postpartum haemorrhage associated with hypotension may cause pituitary necrosis (Sheehan's syndrome) and hence hypopituitarism. This is, however, most uncommon nowadays in developed countries.

Infarction and haemorrhage may occur in pituitary tumours, and the latter may later calcify to cause a pituitary 'stone'. Infarction of pituitary tumours may cause the 'empty sella syndrome', when CSF is present in the pituitary fossa. This can be demonstrated by contrast studies or CT scanning. These patients, however, may have completely normal pituitary function. In addition, severe head trauma may be associated with pituitary insufficiency, including diabetes insipidus, as a result of either hypothalamic damage or interference with hypophyseal portal vascular connections.

The commonest causes of hypopituitarism, however, are pituitary tumours in adults and craniopharyngiomas in children. Isolated anterior pituitary hormonal defects also occur (e.g. isolated growth hormone deficiency), probably related to abnormalities of hypothalamic hormone secretion.

In progressive hypopituitarism there is usually a characteristic order in the development of trophic hormone deficiency. Usually GH and LH secretion fail first, followed later by that of FSH and ACTH and TSH. Prolactin deficiency is rare except in post-partum pituitary necrosis. Diabetes insipidus is extremely uncommon in patients with pituitary tumours.

Patients with hypopituitarism may present in coma. The reasons for this include hypoglycaemia (in part related to the increased insulin sensitivity caused by growth hormone and cortisol deficiency), hypothyroidism, hypothermia and water intoxication. They may have a normochromic anaemia although the pallor of the skin is greater than their degree of anaemia. They are usually of normal weight. The other clinical features of hypopituitarism vary according to the trophic hormone deficiency and the stage of development at which the hypopituitarism develops.

Growth hormone deficiency is an important cause of short stature in children, as well as retarded bone development. There are no clinical features of growth hormone deficiency in adults, but there is increased insulin sensitivity. In children the condition may be either an isolated congenital defect or acquired, most commonly in association with a craniopharyngioma.

Children with congenital growth hormone deficiency have an immature appearance, with fine skin and delicate features (Fig. 2.11). They tend to be fat, of

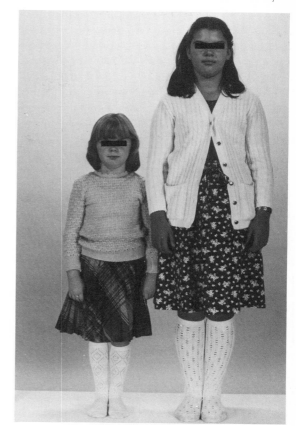

Fig. 2.11 *Two sisters 18 months apart in age. The girl on the left has isolated GH deficiency.*

normal proportions, and are below the third percentile in height. Growth is not entirely absent; children with this condition usually grown about 1cm a year. The cause of the syndrome is unclear. It may be due to decrease in the growth hormone releasing factor, and may occasionally be associated with gonadotrophin deficiency. Early diagnosis is essential; effective treatment with parenteral growth hormone is now available (but recently withdrawn because of the development of Creutzfeld–Jacob disease in a few patients so treated) but the potential for catch-up growth decreases as the child gets older.

Congenital LHRH deficiency occurs (Kallmann's syndrome), which may be associated with anosmia due to an associated abnormality of development of the olfactory lobe. Gonadotrophin deficiency occurs early in progressive hypopituitarism. In adolescents there is normal or increased height due to delayed epiphyseal closure which causes a eunuchoid habitus. In adults there is decreased libido, impotence and a decrease in sperm count; testicular size decreases and the testes become soft. In addition there is loss of pubic, axillary and facial hair, and in women dyspareunia and amenorrhoea, due to decreased oestrogen secretion. Infertility is common in both men and women.

Prolactin deficiency is rare and associated with failure of post-partum lactation.

Undersecretion of TSH in children causes growth retardation. When hypothyroidism develops in adults, the swelling of the subcutaneous tissue is less prominent in secondary hypothyroidism than in the primary form of the disease. ACTH undersecretion is associated with many of the features of primary adrenal insufficiency but aldosterone secretion is normal and in pituitary adrenal insufficiency there is pallor rather than pigmentation of the skin.

ADH deficiency causes diabetes insipidus with polydipsia and polyuria. Cranial diabetes insipidus may occur temporarily after pituitary surgery. Its severity varies and between 4 and 20 litres of dilute urine may be produced over 24 hours. It is rare in patients with untreated pituitary tumours. It is particularly difficult to control if, in the presence of hypothalamic disease, the function of the thirst centre is also abnormal.

Investigation of suspected hypopituitarism should be carried out as detailed on p.34. Before posterior pituitary function is investigated, it is important to replace ACTH and TSH with hydrocortisone and thyroxine if these hormones are deficient, since such deficiency is associated with a decrease in the glomerular filtration rate and this may mask diabetes insipidus.

INVESTIGATION OF PATIENTS WITH PITUITARY DISEASE

Assessment of Pituitary Anatomy

In patients with pituitary disease, both anatomical and physiological aspects of the pituitary have to be considered. Visual fields may be tested by confrontation with a red pin or, more formally, by using either a Bjerrum screen (red and white objects) or the Goldman apparatus (lights of different intensity and colour). The detection of pituitary enlargement depends on radiological investigations and, of these, the most important are the anteroposterior and lateral views of the pituitary fossa (Figs 2.12, 2.13). In the assessment of the lateral skull x-ray, it is important to look at the angulation or rotation of the patient's head; the anterior clinoid processes should be superimposed. Calcification may be seen in the suprasellar region in patients with craniopharyngioma. Calcification is also seen after tuberculous meningitis, with aneurysms of the carotid artery, and with pituitary stones. If there is any reason (from the plain skull x-rays or because of abnormal pituitary function) to suspect a pituitary adenoma, tomography of the fossa can be carried out, using cuts every 2–3 mm because less frequent ones may miss the subtle changes in contour sometimes associated with a microadenoma. This technique may reveal an abnormality in a fossa that was previously thought to be normal. Air encephalography used to be used to define the upper border of a tumour but, because of side-effects, this procedure has been superseded by metrizamide cisternography. Metrizamide, a water-soluble contrast medium, can be introduced by cisternal puncture into the CSF, giving a good outline of the suprasellar region with fewer side-effects than air encephalography.

CT scanning provides a valuable non-invasive means of delineating tumours and has largely superseded the above radiological methods; it is also particularly valuable in delineating lateral extensions of pituitary tumours into the cavernous sinus. Large tumours with suprasellar extensions may also be seen with this technique (Fig. 2.14). More recently, scanners which can reconstruct pictures in either the anteroposterior or lateral planes have become available, providing a non-invasive means of getting a three-dimensional picture of a pituitary tumour (Fig. 2.15).

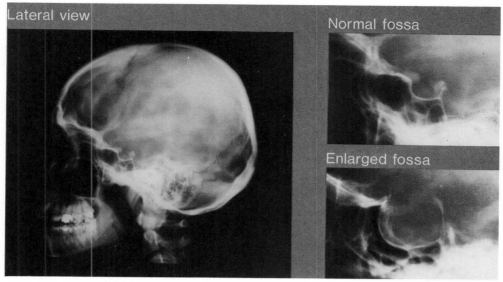

Fig. 2.12 *Investigation of a suspected pituitary tumour should include plain skull x-rays. Large tumours may uniformly expand the fossa and this is called ballooning.*

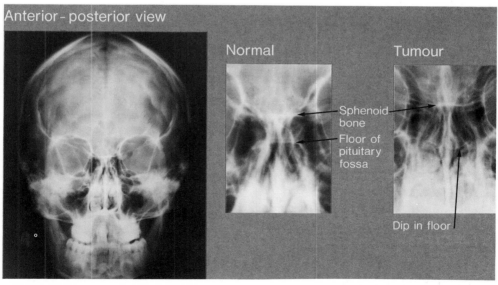

Fig. 2.13 *Anteroposterior views of the skull may be helpful in demonstrating the floor of the pituitary fossa. This is usually flat but, when a tumour is present, there may be a central dip or sloping down of the floor on one side.*

Tumour with suprasellar extension

Tumour with lateral extension

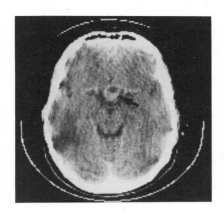

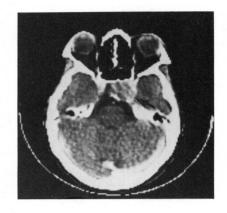

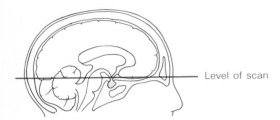

Level of scan

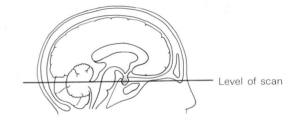

Level of scan

Fig. 2.14 *Computerised tomography of the skull is an important non-invasive method for demonstrating suprasellar and lateral extension of pituitary tumours.*

Assessment of Pituitary Function in Suspected Hypopituitarism

It is essential to assess and correct anterior pituitary function before testing that of the posterior pituitary. This is because cortisol deficiency may decrease the symptoms of diabetes insipidus, in part by decreasing the glomerular filtration rate. Basal hormone levels give a great deal of information and it is therefore important to measure thyroxine, cortisol, prolactin, LH, FSH, TSH, testosterone or oestradiol. It is then important to correlate the levels of effector gland hormone (e.g. thyroxine) with that of the trophic hormone (e.g. TSH). Thus a low thyroxine in the presence of a low TSH implies hypothyroidism due to a central rather than an end-organ deficit. Similar reasoning can be used to assess LH reserve in men by measuring both LH and testosterone.

The insulin stress test is a standard way of assessing ACTH and growth hormone reserves, and is safe if adequate precautions are taken. It should not be done in patients with known ischaemic heart disease or epilepsy (because hypoglycaemia is one of the metabolic causes of epilepsy). Intravenous glucose and hydrocortisone should be at hand, and, throughout the test, patients should not be left unattended. When performing this test, the insulin is given intravenously in a dose of between 0.15 to 0.3 units per kilogram depending on whether there is likely to be any insulin resistance (e.g. in patients with acromegaly or Cush-

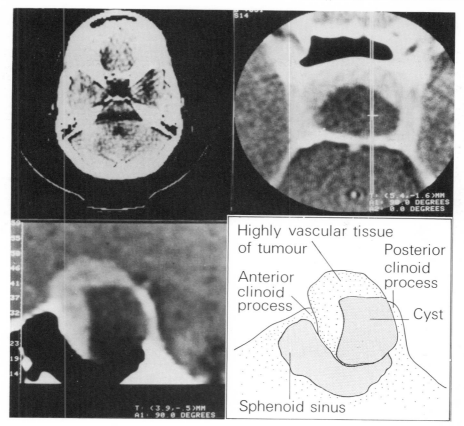

Fig. 2.15 *Computerised tomography of the skull in a patient with a cystic pituitary tumour showing the value of a reconstruction of the sagittal scan of the pituitary region.*

ing's syndrome). Adequate hypoglycaemia has to occur (blood glucose < 2.2 mmol/l) and this should be accompanied by symptoms and signs of neuroglycopenia, e.g. tachycardia and sweating. At intervals during the test, blood samples are taken to measure glucose, cortisol and growth hormone (0, 30, 45, 60, 90 min). Plasma cortisol levels should rise to above 550 nmol/l and growth hormone levels to above 20 mU/l (Fig. 2.16). If the growth hormone does not rise, this implies growth hormone deficiency; if the level of cortisol does not rise, however, this could be due to pituitary insufficiency or primary adrenal failure. This can best be differentiated either by measuring ACTH levels, which are high in primary adrenal failure, or

giving synthetic ACTH intramuscularly and measuring the cortisol response to this.

TRH 200 μg and LHRH 100 μg may be given intravenously to assess the reserves of TSH, LH and FSH. However, these tests are not as useful in pituitary disease as had formerly been hoped and it is probably true that as much information can be obtained from measuring the basal concentrations of the hormones as discussed above.

If insulin-induced hypoglycaemia is contra-indicated, then glucagon (1 mg subcutaneously) may be given as this stimulates both growth hormone and cortisol, though the mechanism by which it does this is unclear. However, it is not such a reliable stimulus of

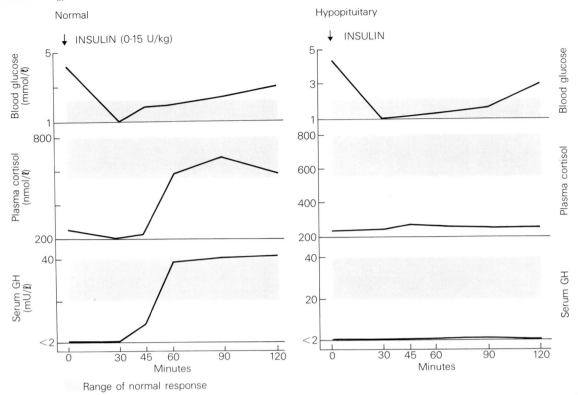

Fig. 2.16 *Insulin stress test in a normal subject and in a patient with hypopituitarism (note the delayed recovery from hypoglycaemia and the impaired cortisol and growth hormone responses).*

these two hormones as is insulin hypoglycaemia. Growth hormone reserve may also be tested by the intravenous administration of arginine.

After assessment and replacement of the anterior pituitary, the function of the posterior pituitary is assessed. If there is polyuria, then plasma and urine osmolality should be measured. If the plasma osmolality is above 300 mosmol/kg and the urine is not concentrated, then diabetes insipidus is extremely likely. If the diagnosis is in doubt, then posterior pituitary function is tested with water deprivation. Other causes of polyuria, including diabetes mellitus and chronic renal failure (caused by osmotic diuretics, glucose and urea), hypercalcaemia (which causes nephrogenic diabetes insipidus because calcium inter-

feres with the action of ADH in the distal tubule), and hypokalaemia must be excluded. During water deprivation, it is important to ensure that the patient is not drinking. This is particularly so in patients with psychogenic polydipsia who have to be carefully differentiated from patients with true diabetes insipidus. Water is withheld for up to 8 hours and during the test urine and plasma osmolality are measured. In normal subjects the urine osmolality should rise above 600 mosmol/kg and there should be little rise in plasma osmolality (Fig. 2.17). Certainly it should not rise above 300 mosmol/kg. At the end of 8 hours if there is no antidiuresis then intranasal or intramuscular vasopressin is given. If the urine then concentrates, the diagnosis is one of cranial diabetes insipidus. If, despite the administration of

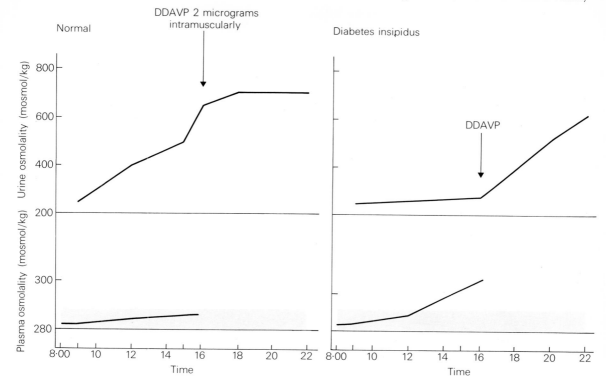

Fig. 2.17 *Water deprivation tests in a normal subject and in a patient with diabetes insipidus (note the impaired ability to concentrate urine, the large rise in urine osmolality after DDAVP and the excessive rise in plasma osmolality).*

vasopressin, no concentration occurs the diagnosis is one of nephrogenic diabetes insipidus.

It is important to note that this test can cause dangerous electrolyte disturbance in patients with severe diabetes insipidus. If the plasma osmolality rises above 300 mosmol/kg or the patient loses greater than 3% of body weight, the test should be stopped, and the patient allowed free access to fluids, and vasopressin administered.

Replacement Therapy in Hypopituitary Patients

In patients who are ACTH deficient, glucocorticoid replacement alone is necessary since mineralocorticoid secretion is not under pituitary control. Hydrocortisone is usually taken twice daily, on waking and in the early evening, usually in a dose of 20 mg and 10 mg (total 30 mg). This drug is given in preference to cortisone acetate which is irregularly absorbed and has to be converted in the liver to cortisol. When using hydrocortisone, it is possible to monitor the levels of cortisol obtained, which is important because the needs of individual patients vary considerably from 15 mg to 60 mg per day. During this procedure the peak level in the morning should be between 850 and 1120 nmol/l and the evening peak should be between 400 and 850 nmol/l. In the presence of ACTH deficiency, patients should carry a steroid card in case of an emergency, as well as a bracelet such as that supplied by the Medicalert organisation.

In the presence of TSH deficiency, thyroxine should be given in a dose of 0.15–0.2 mg daily. It is rarely necessary to exceed this dose. Adequate replacement is indicated by circulating tri-iodothyronine (T_3) in the normal range.

Growth hormone deficiency in children has been treated by twice-weekly injections of purified human growth hormone (see above). Because of possible slow virus contamination this treatment has recently been stopped. It is hoped that biosynthetic growth hormone will soon be available. In the future, such children may be treated with growth hormone releasing factor (GRF), which is easier to synthesise and obtain. It is not necessary to treat GH deficiency in adults.

It is important to treat gonadotrophin deficiency, because long-term sex steroid deficiency will lead to premature osteoporosis. In males, Sustanon or Primoteston, mixtures of testosterone esters with an extended duration of action, may be given intramuscularly in doses of 250–500 mg every 2–4 weeks. This will provide adequate testosterone levels. More recently, oral testosterone derivatives have become available; these provide rather variable testosterone levels without any apparent side-effects (e.g. testosterone undecanoate, 40 mg three times daily). For women with gonadotrophin deficiency it is usual to give oestrogen and cyclical medroxyprogesterone. A typical regime is to give ethinyl oestradiol, 30 μg daily, for four weeks and during the last week to administer medroxyprogesterone, 5 mg daily, after which a withdrawal bleed occurs. While these two therapies result in replacement of deficient steroid hormone production, follicle stimulating hormone and luteinising hormone (both contained in human menopausal gonadotrophin) have to be injected if either spermatogenesis or ovulation are required.

Posterior pituitary replacement is best given with an analogue of vasopressin, although agents that stimulate release of vasopressin or potentiate its action on the kidney are now available for patients with partial vasopressin deficiency. The treatment of diabetes insipidus has been revolutionised by the development of a long-acting analogue of arginine vasopressin. The molecule has been modified so that no vasoconstriction occurs and the diuretic effect is preserved and prolonged. The drug (desmopressin, 1-desamino-8D-arginine-vasopressin: DDAVP), may be given intranasally (5–20 μg), intramuscularly (2 μg) or orally (50–100 μg) once or twice daily according to the needs of the patient. In partial vasopressin deficiency, chlorpropamide, by increasing the sensitivity of the renal tubule to vasopressin, may result in a reduction in urine volume. The usual dose is between 100 and 350 mg daily. Clearly this may cause hypoglycaemia, particularly in the elderly, who should be warned to have some food at bedtime to prevent this. Carbamazepine (200 mg three times daily) has a similar antidiuretic effect.

FUNCTIONING PITUITARY TUMOURS

Prolactinomas

It is now known that prolactin is the commonest hormone to be secreted by pituitary tumours and microadenomas which may be as small as 2–3 mm in diameter occur frequently. Non-secreting pituitary tumours may also cause hyperprolactinaemia by preventing the prolactin inhibiting factor dopamine from reaching normal prolactin-secreting cells. Hypothalamic tumours which compress the pituitary stalk may have the same effect on circulating prolactin levels.

Hyperprolactinaemia in women classically causes galactorrhoea and amenorrhoea, but irregular cycles may occur. Infertility is common because of anovulation, which is caused because prolactin interferes with the action of the gonadotrophins LH and FSH on the ovary as well as by interfering centrally with positive feedback of oestrogen at the hypothalamus and pituitary which normally results in ovulation. Hyperprolactinaemic women may have acne and hirsuties because prolactin increases the secretion of some adrenal androgens. The oestrogen-containing contraceptive preparations increase the number of lactotrophs and may exacerbate hyperprolactinaemia. The contraceptive pill should not therefore be given to women with irregular or absent menstrual cycles.

Galactorrhoea in men is less common than in women. Slight gynaecomastia can occur; this is not, however, typical of hyperprolactinaemia and is more commonly seen in patients with high oestrogen levels. Soft testes may occur in hyperprolactinaemia, and the sperm count and seminal volume may decrease.

Table 2.4

Causes of Hyperprolactinaemia

1. Physiological – sleep, coitus, pregnancy, suckling, neonatal
2. Prolactin-secreting pituitary tumours
   (secreted alone or in combination, e.g. with GH or ACTH)
3. Hypothalamic disorders
4. Pituitary stalk section (e.g. surgical or head injury)
5. Drugs
   a. Dopamine blockers – metoclopramide (Maxolon), sulpiride,
       pimozide, phenothiazines (e.g. chlorpromazine),
       butyrophenones (e.g. haloperidol)
   b. Dopamine depleting agents – reserpine, methyldopa
   c. Miscellaneous – oestrogens (high-dose pill), TRH
6. Hypothyroidism
7. Renal failure
8. Ectopic prolactin secretion
9. Chest wall injury (e.g. trauma, surgery, herpes zoster)

However there may be no abnormal physical signs. Thus patients with so-called psychogenic impotence should not be labelled as such without measurement of serum prolactin and testosterone. In the differential diagnosis of hyperprolactinaemia it is important to exclude other causes, particularly drugs and occult hypothyroidism (see Table 2.4). All causes of hyperprolactinaemia have the same effect on gonadal function. Thus, during lactation post-partum, there is amenorrhoea and infertility, and patients on metoclopramide (given for some gastrointestinal complaints) always have hyperprolactinaemia and this may be associated with gonadal disturbances in both sexes.

Prolactin secretion is best assessed by taking blood samples from unstressed patients. Dynamic function tests, such as giving TRH or metoclopramide, are of little help in the differential diagnosis of an individual patient's problem, even though it is clear that most patients with prolactinomas have an impaired prolactin response to these drugs.

Acromegaly

If growth hormone hypersecretion occurs before fusion of the epiphyses, gigantism results. After fusion, the syndrome of acromegaly often develops over many years and is much commoner than gigantism. Although most commonly associated with eosinophil or acidophil adenomas, it is now recognised that acromegaly can occur with chromophobe adenomas of the pituitary gland. In addition, more rarely, acromegaly can be seen in association with carcinoid tumours of either the lung or pancreas, which secrete growth hormone releasing factor (GRF), thus causing acromegaly by stimulation of the pituitary rather than a primary pituitary tumour.

Acromegaly is a disease that affects nearly all body tissues. Thus all the organs including the viscera and the skin increase in volume, the only exceptions being the brain and spinal cord. The disease progresses so slowly that many years may pass before the victim or friends become aware of the widespread changes that have occurred in appearance and health. Early diagnosis therefore requires a high index of suspicion by all doctors. If necessary old photographs should be consulted in order to decide whether a change has occurred in the patient's appearance (Fig. 2.18). Early diagnosis is important because acromegaly is associated with considerable morbidity and an increased mortality, usually from cardiovascular complications of hypertension or diabetes mellitus.

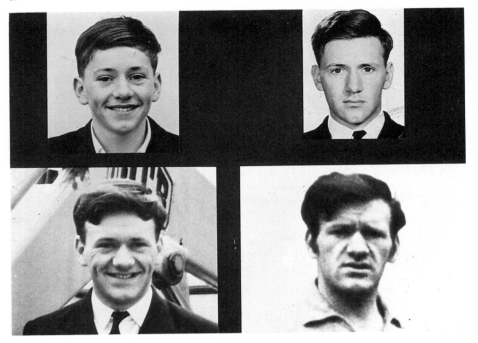

Fig. 2.18 *Sequential photographs demonstrating the development of acromegaly. The changes in the nose and the jaw are particularly obvious.*

The symptoms of the disease may be divided into three groups. There are those that result from the clinical and metabolic effects of excessive growth hormone secretion, particularly increased protein synthesis and insulin antagonism; those which result from local effects of the pituitary tumour; and lastly the endocrine effects of interference with other normal pituitary function.

The clinical effects of excessive growth hormone are numerous. The first change is usually coarsening of the facial features (Fig. 2.19), and acral overgrowth is seen in all patients; both soft tissues and bones enlarge. This is recognised by the patient through a change in appearance and a need for larger rings, gloves and shoes. Enlargement of the facial bones is most striking in the mandible where there is prognathism and increased interdental separation (Fig. 2.20). The supra-orbital ridges and zygomatic bones also enlarge, macroglossia

occurs, and increased sweating also occurs in about 80% of patients with active acromegaly. Other skin changes are apparent; fibromata mollusca occur frequently and increased sebaceous activity has been noted which causes an apparently greasy skin. In addition, hirsuties may appear in women, and 40% of patients gain weight. The ribs and costal cartilages enlarge, and in long-standing cases this leads to a barrel chest. Cartilaginous proliferation of the larynx, together with large sinuses, frequently results in a deep, resonant voice. In the cardiovascular system, hypertension occurs frequently. Occasionally, patients have a coexistent phaeochromocytoma or a Conn (aldosterone-secreting) tumour as part of a multiple endocrine disorder, but in most patients the hypertension is idiopathic. Cardiomyopathy may occur in association with acromegaly. In the respiratory system, there is often thickening of the mucous membranes, and

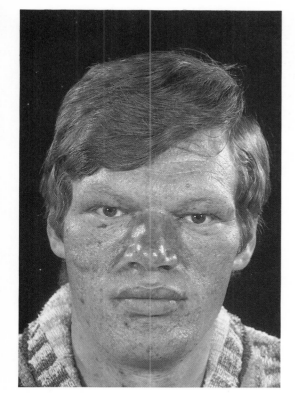

Fig. 2.19 *Typical appearance of a patient with acromegaly.*

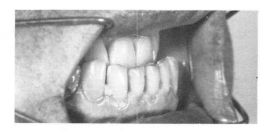

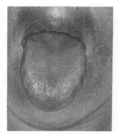 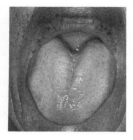

Fig. 2.20 *Prognathism, interdental separation and macroglossia in acromegaly. (Normal tongue on left.)*

sinusitis is frequent. Myopathy may occur as well as peripheral neuropathy so that paraesthesiae in the hands are not always due to carpal tunnel compression (although this is the commonest cause). Another important feature of acromegaly is arthritis. Early osteoarthritis may occur, particularly of the weight-bearing joints (hips and knees); and this can cause great morbidity.

A large number of female patients present with disturbances of the menstrual cycle; most commonly, secondary amenorrhoea occurs. This may be due to a decreased LH reserve as a result of a progressively enlarging pituitary tumour causing hypopituitarism. Hyperprolactinaemia is, however, common in these patients, and this is the most frequent cause of menstrual disturbances and the sometimes-associated galactorrhoea. Men often complain of loss of libido and potency and this, too, frequently relates to associated hyperprolactinaemia.

There are a number of other important endocrine disturbances associated with untreated acromegaly; the most important of these is diabetes mellitus, which occurs in about 30% of patients. Growth hormone causes insulin antagonism and hence increases insulin secretion; this prolonged stimulation eventually leads to β-cell exhaustion and impaired carbohydrate tolerance. A few patients have hypercalcaemia, usually associated with parathyroid adenoma or hyperplasia. Hypercalciuria is seen in about 70% of acromegalics, which may be due to increased concentrations of 1,25-dihydroxy-vitamin D as this is known to rise during physiological states of increased calcium demand, including growth. Goitre, which is often multinodular, is also seen with increased frequency in patients with acromegaly.

The diagnosis of acromegaly is made biochemically with a glucose tolerance test, during which samples for blood glucose and growth hormone are taken. Growth hormone levels should suppress, between 90–180 minutes after oral glucose, to < 1.0 mU/l (Fig. 2.21). In acromegaly, however, there is either no suppression, partial suppression or even a rise in circulating growth hormone. Growth hormone levels correlate poorly with the clinical picture and are often very high in the youngest patients.

Normal subject

Acromegalic subject

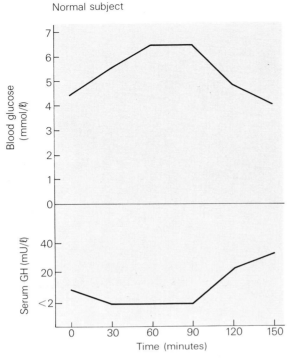
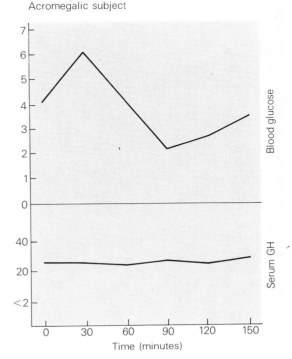

Fig. 2.21 *Growth hormone secretion during an oral glucose tolerance test in a normal subject and in a patient with acromegaly (note failure of growth hormone to suppress during the test).*

Cushing's Disease

The hypersecretion of ACTH by a pituitary tumour leads to bilateral adrenocortical hyperplasia and hence Cushing's syndrome. Pituitary-dependent Cushing's syndrome is known as Cushing's disease, and is discussed in Chapter 4.

Other Tumours

Very rarely, tumours of the pituitary secreting TSH may produce hyperthyroidism. Gonadotrophin-producing tumours are probably more common and may be missed in menopausal patients where gonadotrophin levels would be expected to be high.

THE TREATMENT OF NON-FUNCTIONING PITUITARY TUMOURS

For small non-functioning tumours (microadenomas) of less than 10 mm in diameter, a policy of observation is usually satisfactory. Pituitary function should be assessed in these patients and they should have yearly skull x-rays and assessment of visual fields to decide if any change in size is occurring. If they do enlarge, patients should be recommended for treatment. This may be done surgically by the trans-sphenoidal or transfrontal routes or by using various forms of interstitial or external irradiation. Drugs such as bromocriptine may shrink prolactin-secreting pituitary tumours but are not used for non-functioning tumours.

Surgery (Fig. 2.22)

Transfrontal surgery has a greater morbidity and mortality than trans-sphenoidal surgery. The main indication for the former is decompression of the optic chiasm in patients with a large suprasellar extension (greater than 1 cm). Surgery using this route virtually never results in complete removal of the tumour; subsequent radiotherapy is necessary and important as a considerable proportion of the tumours recur. Trans-sphenoidal surgery for pituitary tumours obtains the best results if the tumour is small. This technique, during which it may be possible to dissect the pituitary adenoma from the rest of the normal pituitary using an operating microscope, clearly requires a great deal of expertise but is increasingly widely applied. The trans-sphenoidal route has a low morbidity and mortality but may not always be feasible in patients with big lateral extensions of their tumour, or a very large suprasellar extension. However, many neurosurgeons now use the trans-sphenoidal route to decompress patients with moderate sized suprasellar extensions. Complications include CSF rhinorrhoea, sinusitis and meningitis, but these are uncommon. Diabetes insipidus may also occur, due to hypothalamic damage, but this is usually temporary. After surgery it is important to reassess pituitary function because a proportion of patients become hypopituitary.

Radiotherapy

Radiotherapy has been used for many years in the treatment of pituitary tumours. Most experience has been gained with the linear accelerator and cobalt machines. Prior to treatment the tumour has to be adequately delineated in all its aspects. Treatment usually takes five weeks and, if carefully carried out, has no major side-effects but hypopituitarism may develop some years later.

THE TREATMENT OF FUNCTIONING PITUITARY TUMOURS

The treatment of functioning tumours of the pituitary depends on a number of factors: the severity of the

Transfrontal route   Trans-sphenoidal routes

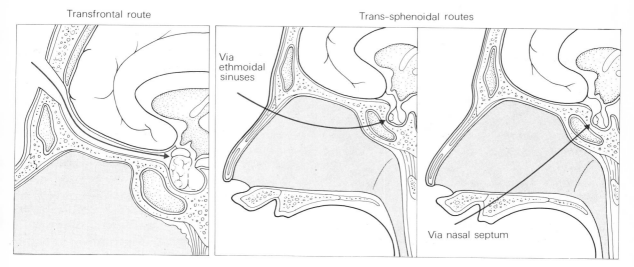

Via ethmoidal sinuses

Via nasal septum

Fig. 2.22 *The different approaches to the pituitary fossa used during surgery for pituitary tumours.*

symptoms; the presence of complications; and the hormonal levels. The type of treatment and expertise that are available will of necessity also have an important bearing on the advice given to the patient.

Treatment of any functioning pituitary tumour should aim to produce normal hormone levels, and to improve the clinical and metabolic abnormalities associated with these, without any side-effects, including hypopituitarism. Unfortunately all currently available treatments have their problems and there is at present no ideal management of any of the pituitary hypersecretory syndromes.

Prolactinomas

Small pituitary tumours secreting prolactin may be successfully treated with bromocriptine, a long-acting dopamine agonist which suppresses prolactin levels. This drug is usually given in a dose of 7.5 mg daily (2.5 mg three times daily with food). In women, when the prolactin levels are suppressed the menstrual pattern returns usually within 2 or 3 months. This is associated with ovular cycles and a return of fertility. In men, potency is usually restored if gonadotrophin secretion is unaffected. When bromocriptine is used in the treatment of infertility, it does not appear to be teratogenic, but it is usually stopped at the beginning of pregnancy. The long-term effects of taking bromocriptine over a number of years are not clear at present, but patients treated for 14 years have not, so far, developed complications. However, care should be used in administering this drug to patients with pituitary tumours, especially macroadenomas, who wish to become pregnant because the pituitary may enlarge during pregnancy and cause chiasmal compression. In the presence of a pituitary tumour, therefore, it is important to treat the tumour in its own right (with either surgery or radiotherapy) prior to embarking on pregnancy.

Side-effects of bromocriptine may occur but are not frequently a problem if the drug is started slowly and taken during food. Early in treatment, nausea and dizziness due to postural hypotension (the drug is also an α-receptor agonist) may occur. These side-effects usually disappear with time or if the drug dosage is temporarily slightly reduced.

Large tumours associated with high prolactin secre-

tion must be treated in their own right, either with surgery, radiotherapy or a combination of the two. In addition, there are now good animal data to suggest that bromocriptine may decrease the size of pituitary tumours secreting prolactin by decreasing DNA turnover in the lactotrophs. Prospective trials have shown that bromocriptine decreases pituitary tumour size in over 60% of patients receiving it alone. Thus, in the presence of large tumours, even those causing local pressure symptoms, bromocriptine can be used provided careful monitoring of the visual fields and visual acuity is carried out. If these worsen or do not improve on the drug then surgery is indicated because the longer there is pressure on the optic chiasm the less reversible is the consequent field defect. The use of bromocriptine in the treatment of large prolactin-secreting tumours may either make surgery easier (if the tumour decreases in size) or obviate the need for surgery entirely.

Acromegaly

Small tumours which are not causing local pressure effects can be treated with either conventional radiotherapy or surgery. Treatment is important because acromegaly decreases life expectancy.

Conventional radiotherapy is widely available and effective but unfortunately the beneficial effects may take some years to develop. However, when carefully carried out 80% of patients have growth hormone levels below 10 mU/l ten years after treatment. Trans-sphenoidal removal of the pituitary tumour may cure acromegalic patients, and this is particularly true of those with small pituitary tumours. Clearly the effects on GH are rapid. Patients with large tumours are less frequently cured because it is more difficult to remove the whole tumour, and hypopituitarism is more frequent after surgery in these patients.

Recently bromocriptine has been found to be effective in the treatment of acromegaly. It has already been mentioned that, in normal subjects, dopamine causes a rise in circulating growth hormone. In acromegaly, however, there is a paradoxical fall in serum growth hormone in patients given drugs which stimulate dopamine receptors. Bromocriptine may be given in doses between 20 and 60 mg daily (taken 6-hourly in divided doses). On this treatment there is a significant growth hormone reduction in 70% of patients, and over 90% notice an improvement in one or more of their clinical symptoms. In only 20% of patients, however, do growth hormone levels become normal.

Provided it is started slowly, the initiating side-effects of nausea and vomiting are not a problem. In the long-term, using these higher doses, constipation may develop, but this is not usually troublesome.

Bromocriptine therapy is indicated in patients who have not yet responded to radiotherapy or in whom growth hormone levels are not reduced to normal after surgery. Rarely, it is used as sole treatment in elderly patients with complications of acromegaly or in others unwilling to undergo other forms of pituitary therapy.

After successful treatment of acromegaly, glucose tolerance improves, as does hypertension; sweating decreases, facial appearances improve, and hand and foot size decrease.

Large growth hormone-secreting tumours have to be treated in their own right, either with surgery, radiotherapy or a combination of the two. A small proportion of growth hormone-secreting tumours decrease in size on bromocriptine treatment, but this effect is less dramatic than with prolactin-secreting tumours.

Cushing's Disease

Pituitary-dependent Cushing's disease in children responds well to external radiotherapy, but this treatment is of little value for adults. Trans-sphenoidal surgery, with selective removal of an adenoma, probably offers the best chance of curing this condition. If bilateral adrenalectomy is performed, then pituitary irradiation should also be given to prevent the development of Nelson's syndrome (i.e. postadrenalectomy hyperpigmentation with a pituitary tumour).

3

The Thyroid Gland

DEVELOPMENT AND ANATOMY

The thyroid is formed in the first month of fetal development from the floor of the pharynx between the first and the second branchial pouches. The thyroglossal duct originates in the midline at the junction of the anterior two-thirds and posterior one-third of the tongue (foramen caecum) and migrates to the anterior part of the neck. This duct is subsequently obliterated, but fragments can persist as cysts or form sites of ectopic thyroid tissue (lingual thyroid, or pyramidal lobe close to the isthmus), or result in a retrosternal thyroid due to excessive descent.

The adult thyroid consists of two lateral lobes joined by a central isthmus lying anterior to the trachea

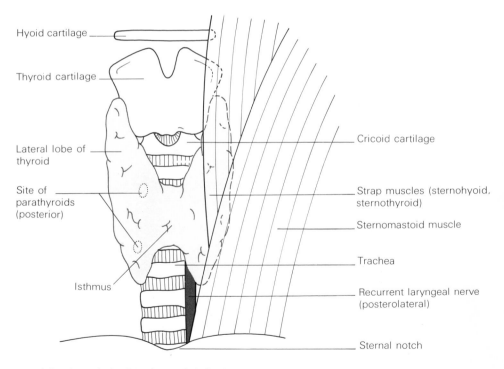

Fig. 3.1 *Position of the thyroid gland in the neck indicating relationship to surrounding structures.*

Hyoid cartilage

Thyroid cartilage

Lateral lobe of thyroid

Site of parathyroids (posterior)

Isthmus

Cricoid cartilage

Strap muscles (sternohyoid, sternothyroid)

Sternomastoid muscle

Trachea

Recurrent laryngeal nerve (posterolateral)

Sternal notch

opposite the fifth, sixth and seventh cervical vertebrae (Fig. 3.1). It is bound to the trachea and the isthmus usually covers the second and third tracheal rings. It may be palpated by standing behind the patient and curling the middle three fingers round the medial border of the sternomastoid muscles just above the sternal notch so that the tips of the fingers rest on the trachea. The lateral lobes are normally soft and conical, thicker at the lower pole and tapering to the upper pole. The gland moves with the trachea under the palpating fingers when the patient swallows. Nevertheless, a normal gland may not be palpable in 75% of men and 50% of women depending on their build and the bulk of the neck. Any enlargement of the gland is known as a goitre. Estimates of the size of the gland by volume or weight, on clinical examination, are notoriously inaccurate. The most widely adopted criterion of a goitre is a thyroid whose lateral lobes have a volume greater than the terminal phalanges of the thumbs of the person being examined. A thyroid that is visible as well as palpable is almost always enlarged.

Histology

The thyroid is composed of numerous functional units or follicles separated by connective tissue (Fig. 3.2). In the connective tissue are parafollicular or C-cells which have a separate origin from the thyroid and secrete calcitonin. Each thyroid follicle is spherical and lined with epithelial cells surrounding a central colloid-containing space. The size of the follicles varies considerably, but in general the height of the follicular cells is inversely related to the amount of colloid. The nucleus of each follicular cell is close to the base, which is the outer surface adjacent to the capillary, and the apex consists of microvilli pointing into the colloid.

THYROID HORMONE FORMATION AND RELEASE

The thyroid produces two major hormones, tri-iodothyronine (T_3) and thyroxine (T_4). These are synthesised in the thyroid follicles in a series of complicated steps, stored in the colloid as part of thyroglobulin and

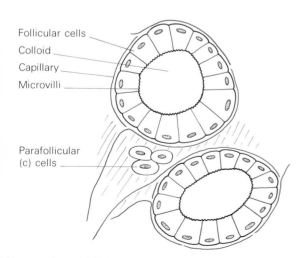

Fig. 3.2 *Thyroid follicles and parafollicular (c) cells.*

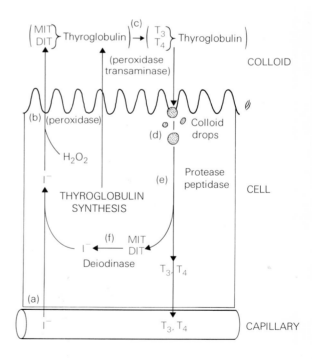

(a) Iodide transport (b) Oxidation (c) Coupling
(d) Colloid resorption (e) Proteolysis (f) Deiodination

Fig. 3.3 *Thyroid hormone synthesis and release.*

released from the follicle cells into the circulation where they are largely bound to serum proteins (Fig. 3.3). A small proportion is unbound or 'free'. It is the free hormones that govern the body's metabolic state by their action on a wide variety of peripheral cells.

Hormone synthesis

Iodine in the diet (in drinking water and food such as fish or iodised bread or salt) is wholly absorbed from the gut and about 150 μg are required daily. Inorganic iodide (I^-) is concentrated in the thyroid follicles by active transport across the cell membrane (the iodide trap) and rapidly transferred across the cell into the colloid lumen. During this process, iodide is oxidised by peroxidase and linked to tyrosine molecules to form mono-iodotyrosines (MIT) and di-iodotyrosines (DIT) which are not metabolically active (Fig. 3.4). The tyrosines which are not iodinated are contained within

thyroglobulin which is a large protein, synthesised by the follicular cells and secreted into the lumen. MIT and DIT within thyroglobulin are then coupled by further enzyme action (transaminase, peroxidase) to form thyroxine (T_4) and tri-iodothyronine (T_3), still linked with thyroglobulin and stored in the lumen.

Hormone release

Thyroxine and tri-iodothyronine linked to thyroglobulin are reabsorbed into the follicular cells in colloid drops by endocytosis. T_4 and T_3 are then separated from the thyroglobulin by proteases contained within lyso-zomes. Any uncoupled MIT and DIT are further de-iodinated to release tyrosine and iodide which may be available for recycling. T_4 and T_3 are then secreted into the circulation, where they are largely bound to circulating plasma proteins. Thyroxine binding globulin (TBG) has the greatest affinity for T_4 and a lower affinity

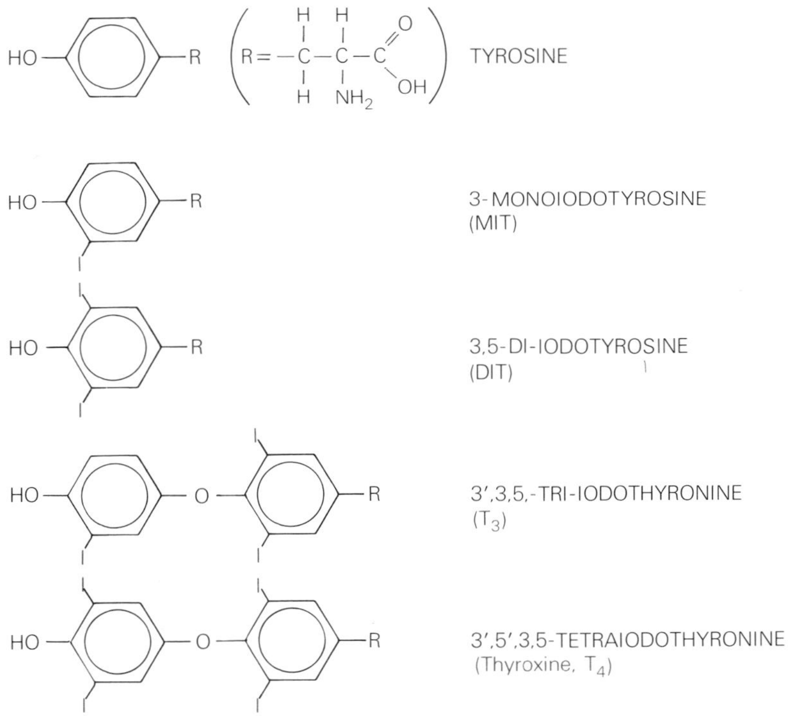

Fig. 3.4 *Structures of iodotyrosines and iodothyronines.*

for T_3, although a small proportion of these hormones also binds to pre-albumin and, to a lesser extent, albumin.

Measurement of circulating hormone

Measurement of total thyroid hormones includes protein-bound and free fractions. Concentration of total T_4 in normal serum lies between 50 and 140 nmol/l, whereas the free fraction lies between 9 and 24 pmol/l. The concentration of total T_3 lies between 1 and 3 nmol/l and the free fraction between 5 and 10 pmol/l. Alterations in the concentration of serum proteins will affect total T_4 and total T_3 levels. Such changes in proteins may result in misleading elevation or reduction of total thyroxine and tri-iodothyronine. This can be recognised either by direct measurement of TBG, to arrive at a T_4/TBG ratio, or by an indirect method of estimating the available binding sites for thyroid hormone. Radio-isotope-labelled T_3 and a resin able to bind T_3 is mixed with the serum of the patient and a proportion of the label will become attached to serum proteins according to the number of binding sites available. The percentage of radio-isotope bound to the resin can then be used to derive a free thyroxine index:

$$FTI = total\ T_4 \times \frac{T_3\ resin\ uptake}{100}$$

Techniques which measure free fractions of T_4 or T_3 are not usually influenced by the amount of TBG present.

Whilst T_4 is produced entirely by the thyroid, T_3 is also produced by peripheral conversion from T_4 in cells of the kidney, liver, heart, anterior pituitary and other tissues. T_4 is deiodinated to the active metabolite T_3 or an inactive metabolite reverse T_3 (rT_3) (Fig. 3.5). The mechanism controlling these conversions is poorly understood. In healthy individuals, T_4 is largely converted to T_3 but in severely ill people suffering from a variety of acute or chronic illnesses, less T_3 and more reverse T_3 is produced.

CONTROL OF THYROID FUNCTION

In normal individuals, the synthesis and release of thyroid hormones is regulated by thyroid stimulating hormone (TSH) released from the anterior pituitary. TSH is a glycoprotein consisting of alpha and beta subunits linked by noncovalent bonds. The alpha subunit is similar to that found in three other glycoprotein hormones (LH, FSH, HCG) but the beta subunits differ (see Chapter 1). Isolated subunits do not show activity but combine to form biologically active units. TSH is in turn regulated by thyrotrophin releasing hormone (TRH) from the hypothalamus. TRH is a tripeptide which

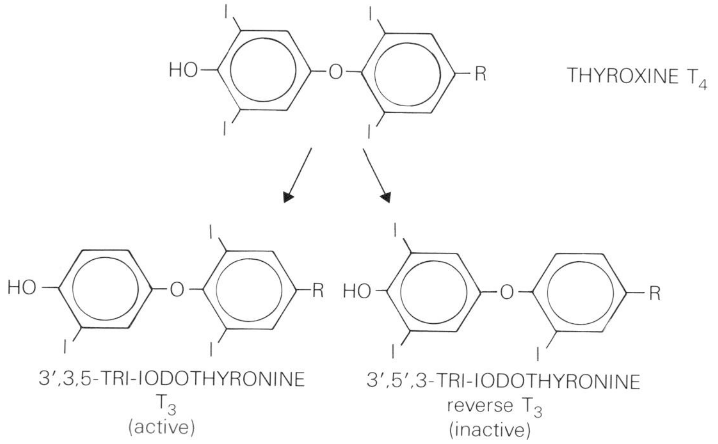

Fig. 3.5 *Deiodination of thyroxine to tri-iodothyronine (T_3) or reverse T_3.*

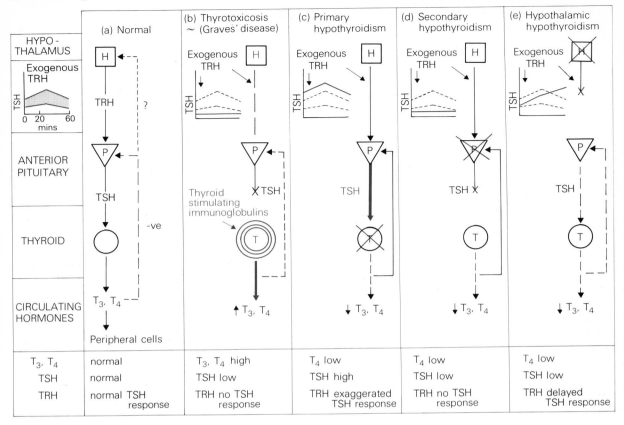

Fig. 3.6 *Control of thyroid function and results of thyroid function tests in different types of thyroid disease.*

has been synthesised and is available for exogenous administration. A 200-microgram bolus of TRH given intravenously produces a rise in TSH with a peak at 20 minutes (4–25 mU/l) which falls but does not reach baseline by 60 minutes after injection (Fig. 3.6). A more prolonged effect is produced by oral administration of larger doses of TRH. These doses of TRH are pharmacological. Little is known of the physiology of TRH secretion because it is very difficult to measure.

The levels of circulating T_4 and T_3 exert a feedback effect on the secretion of TSH and possibly TRH. A fall in T_4 and T_3 stimulates TSH release and increase of T_4 and T_3 suppresses TSH (Fig. 3.6a). Conversion of T_4 to T_3 can occur in the anterior pituitary, and this process may govern the secretion of TSH. Normal circulating levels

of TSH range from 0 to 6 mU/l in most commonly used radioimmunoassays. Recent advances in assay methodology have improved the sensitivity of the TSH assay and redefined the lower limit of the normal range.

In the hyperthyroid state, with high circulating thyroid hormone levels, TSH secretion is suppressed and the TSH response to exogenous TRH is absent (Fig. 3.6b). In primary thyroid failure, low levels of circulating thyroid hormones stimulate TSH secretion and the TSH response to TRH is exaggerated (Fig. 3.6c). In pituitary failure, the output of TSH is reduced and circulating hormone levels fall and there may be no TSH response to exogenous TRH (Fig. 3.6d). In hypothalamic disease, endogenous TRH secretion is reduced, resulting in low TSH production and low circulating thyroid hormone levels but the pituitary is still capable of responding, albeit sluggishly, to exogenous TSH and the 60-minute value for TSH is often higher than the 20-minute value (Fig. 3.6e).

Peripheral Effects of Thyroid Hormones

Thyroid hormones play an important role in growth and the regulation of protein, lipid, carbohydrate and mineral metabolism, and greatly affect the rate of oxygen consumption in mammals. Increasing thyroid hormone activity increases amino acid and electrolyte transport into cells, nucleoprotein synthesis, and the activities of tissue enzymes. A decrease in thyroid hormones reduces these activities.

Free thyroid hormones enter cells and bind to specific receptor sites in the cell nuclei. After binding to the nuclear receptor, T_3 induces the formation of a variety of species of messenger RNA coding for proteins such as growth hormones and various enzymes which stimulate lipid formation and lipolysis. Although the primary actions of the thyroid hormones are probably at the nuclear level the major cellular effects are mediated via the mitochondria, which regulate energy production by oxidative phosphorylation. Energy liberated by the oxidation of a substance is transformed into the utilisable high-energy phosphate bonds of adenosine triphosphate (ATP). The system is self-regulatory and the rate of output of ATP controls the rate of oxygen consumption and oxidation of substances. The effects of thyroid hormones on this system are complicated. Physiological and pharmacological levels of thyroid hormones can have very different effects. Small increments in thyroid hormone levels in experimental situations enhance the oxidative process, whereas larger supplements may uncouple oxidative phosphorylation and lead to energy production by alternative and less efficient pathways. The overall effect of thyroid hormones can be determined by the measurement of basal metabolic rate, but this is a cumbersome procedure which is little used in practice nowadays. Hypothyroidism results in a low basal metabolic rate and hyperthyroidism leads to an increased basal metabolic rate. Unfortunately effective tests of peripheral thyroid hormone action are lacking in clinical practice.

Effects of Iodine

Moderate to severe iodine deficiency leads to reduced iodine concentration in the gland, an increase in the proportion of MIT to DIT (see Fig. 3.4), and of T_3 to T_4 with a decrease in serum T_4 and, in severe cases, an increase in TSH. Serum T_3 may remain in the normal range, even in severe iodine deficiency, despite low T_4 indicating preferential secretion of T_3. Chronic iodine deficiency leads to the development of goitre and hypothyroidism and, in children born to iodine deficient mothers, there is a high incidence of impaired brain development.

Iodine excess produces variable effects. Small amounts given acutely do not influence iodine uptake but with large doses, inhibition of organification occurs (Wolf–Chaikoff effect) possibly by inhibition of peroxidase catalysed reactions. Inhibition by an acute large dose of iodide is only a transient phenomenon as the thyroid escapes from inhibition after a few days. This effect is of practical importance in that iodine-containing contrast media used in radiological procedures may temporarily lower thyroid hormone levels and result in misleading tests of thyroid function. Suppression of thyroid function by the administration of potassium iodide before surgery can only be used for a few days. Chronic iodide excess is rarely encountered but can occur in patients taking, long-term, large doses of proprietary iodine-containing cough mixtures which may result in altered organification leading to hypothyroidism and goitre.

Radio-iodine Uptake Studies

Radio-isotopes of iodine (^{123}I, ^{131}I and ^{132}I) are rapidly concentrated in the thyroid and the proportion of a known tracer dose taken up by the gland after a given time can be used as a measure of thyroid function. Such studies are time-consuming and have largely been superseded by direct measurement of thyroid hormones for the determination of thyroid status. Isotope scans are still useful for mapping the size and the position of the thyroid and detecting areas of functioning (hot) and non-functioning (cold) nodules, and for the elucidation of certain defects of thyroid hormone synthesis. Thyroid autonomy may also be demonstrated by failure of suppression of radio-iodine uptake after a course of T_3 (60 μg daily in divided doses for ten days), which would normally reduce the radio-iodine uptake by at least 50%. This test involves giving exogenous T_3 to patients who may already be thyrotoxic, and for this reason has fallen out of favour. The TRH test is now widely used instead of the T_3 suppression test, a lack of TSH response to TRH indicating excess circulating thyroid hormone levels (Fig. 3.6b), but the results of the two tests do not always correlate well, as they are testing different aspects of the thyroid/pituitary axis. Radio-iodine uptake before and after stimulation with exogenous TSH (10 units intramuscularly for three days) may be used to demonstrate thyroid tissue which has been dormant, e.g. hypothyroidism secondary to pituitary disease, or normal thyroid tissue suppressed by a hot nodule, but such tests are rarely necessary. Radio-iodine uptake is negligible in the rare iodine-trapping defects, but is usually increased in organification defects. In the latter, radio-iodine accumulates in the cell but is not incorporated into tyrosine and is rapidly discharged after administration of perchlorate. Perchlorate discharges any radio-iodine left in the form of iodide, normally a negligible fraction of the total radio-iodine accumulated in the labelling process.

Technetium is trapped but not organified by the thyroid and its radio-isotope, ^{99}Tc, can be used instead of radio-iodine to measure thyroid uptake and for thyroid scans. It must be given intravenously and the uptake is usually measured after 20 minutes. It has the advantage of rapidity and lower exposure to radiation by the patient.

DISEASES OF THE THYROID

Iodine deficiency is the major cause of disordered thyroid function worldwide, particularly in mountainous regions, and leads to the formation of goitre and hypothyroidism. In non iodine-deficient areas, autoimmune disorders are believed to be the main cause of thyroid dysfunction. Hyperthyroidism is at one end of the spectrum and hypothyroidism at the other, with various degrees of impaired thyroid function

in-between. Autoimmunity is indicated by the presence of antibodies directed against various components of the thyroid cell. Microsomal antibodies and thyroglobulin antibodies, measured by tanned red cell techniques, are most commonly detected in clinical practice. Presence of these antibodies reflects an underlying autoimmune process but does not necessarily mean that they are the cause of the disorder. Antibodies which bind to the cell surface may stimulate or inhibit thyroid function. There is an association between autoimmune thyroid disease and other organ-specific autoimmune disorders such as pernicious anaemia and diabetes mellitus. Thyroid disease also tends to run in families who share a common genetic predisposition to the development of thyroid dysfunction. Women are much more commonly affected than men and it is not uncommon to find mother and daughter similarly affected, or sisters, one of whom has hyperthyroidism and the other hypothyroidism.

HYPERTHYROIDISM

Hyperthyroidism, or thyrotoxicosis, is due to an excess of the circulating thyroid hormones T_3 and usually T_4. Most cases are either due to Graves' disease which is associated with a diffuse goitre, or due to uninodular or multinodular goitre. Hyperthyroidism may also result from excess thyroxine administered by a doctor (iatrogenic) or by the patient (thyrotoxicosis factitia). Rarely, excess endogenous thyroid hormone may be secreted by metastatic thyroid carcinoma or struma ovarii. Excess TSH-like material (probably human chorionic gonadotrophin, which has a weak affinity for the TSH receptor) leading to hyperthyroidism may be produced by choriocarcinomas or hydatidiform moles or embryonal testicular carcinomas (see Chapter 8). Pituitary tumours primarily secreting TSH are extremely rare and do not justify the routine measurement of serum TSH in patients with thyrotoxicosis. Transient exacerbation of hyperthyroidism may follow therapeutic doses of radio-iodine and may also occur in subacute thyroiditis. Hyperthyroidism may also be unmasked by the administration of iodine (Jod–Basedow phenomenon).

Aetiology of Graves' disease

Graves' disease is believed to be due to circulating thyroid stimulating immunoglobulins (TSI) which bind to the TSH receptors on the thyroid cell and produce prolonged stimulation of cell function (Fig. 3.7). The nomenclature governing these abnormal immunoglobulins is confusing owing to the variety of techniques used in their detection. Serum of patients with Graves' disease given to guinea-pigs or mice whose thyroid glands have been pre-labelled with radio-iodine can cause prolonged stimulation of radio-iodine release, hence the original term long-acting thyroid stimulator (LATS). Such activity is not always demonstrable in the serum of patients with Graves' disease, perhaps due to species differences. LATS activity may be absorbed by human thyroid extract and other sera may inhibit this absorption, i.e. protect LATS from absorption, hence LATS-protector (LATS-p) (Fig. 3.7a). Other techniques demonstrate that immunoglobulins found in patients with Graves' disease inhibit the binding of labelled TSH to the thyroid membrane (thyroid binding inhibiting

immunoglobulin, TBII). Binding to membranes does not necessarily indicate stimulation, which can be demonstrated by measurement of cyclic AMP production or colloid droplet formation or production of T_3 from thyroid cells (Fig. 3.7b). These techniques are important in understanding the mechanisms of Graves' disease but are not routinely available for clinical diagnosis. Separate immunoglobulins may be responsible for the ophthalmic features of Graves' disease. Such immunoglobulins are not usually found in patients with hyperthyroidism due to nodular goitre.

Clinical Features

Hyperthyroidism affects approximately 2% of women in the population; it can occur at any age but is most common in the fourth/fifth decades and is at least ten times more common in women than in men. In overt hyperthyroidism, the patient typically complains of increased irritability, excessive sweating and heat intolerance, weight loss despite a good appetite and

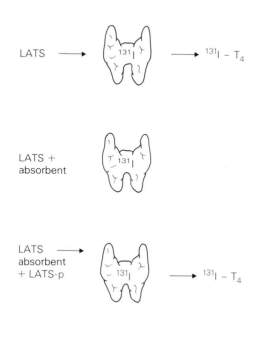

(a)

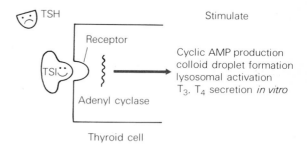

(b)

Fig. 3.7 *Action of thyroid stimulating immunoglobulins (for details see text).*

general fatigue. Patients may also complain of prominent eyes, palpitations, dyspnoea, increased frequency of bowel action and oligomenorrhoea or amenorrhoea. A family history of thyroid disease is often positive.

On examination, the patient appears agitated and the eyes staring due to eyelid retraction. The upper eyelid movement lags behind downward movement of the eye (lid lag). Tremor of the hands is an unreliable sign as it is often present in agitated people who are not thyrotoxic. The skin is warm and moist, the pulse fast or irregular due to atrial fibrillation, and occasionally frank heart failure is present. Proximal myopathy is demonstrated by the patient's difficulty in rising unaided from a sitting or squatting position.

A goitre is usually but not invariably palpable. A solitary nodule or multinodular goitre may be found, but in Graves' disease the goitre is typically diffuse and a bruit may be audible on auscultation.

The eye signs of Graves' disease include periorbital oedema, congested conjunctivae (chemosis), lid retraction, exophthalmos and ophthalmoplegia due to swelling and shortening of the extraocular muscles opposing the limited direction of movement of the eye (Fig. 3.8).

Limitation of upward gaze is one of the earlier features of ophthalmoplegia which, in its more severe form, may cause diplopia and limitation of eye movement in all directions. Rarely, congestive ophthalmopathy may be so severe as to cause pain in the eye, papilloedema or oedema of the macula, leading to deterioration in visual acuity (malignant exophthalmos). Failure of closure of the eyelids may result in keratitis of the exposed cornea.

Other features of Graves' disease include the development of thickened patches of purplish-red skin, usually on the feet or tibia (pretibial myxoedema; present in about 5% of cases), and acropachy with subperiosteal new bone formation and clubbing of the fingers (0.5%). These extrathyroidal manifestations are not found with nodular goitre. Prolonged hyperthyroidism may lead to osteoporosis. Rare associations include hypercalcaemia and myasthenia gravis.

Florid Graves' disease is not difficult to recognise, but lesser degrees of hyperthyroidism may be difficult to distinguish from an anxiety state *per se*. Hyperthyroidism in children causes behavioural changes and may produce a premature growth spurt. In the elderly,

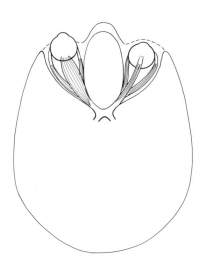

(a) Unilateral exophthalmos swelling of left superior rectus muscle

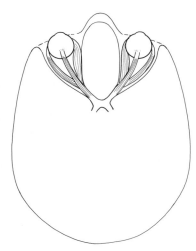

(b) Bilateral exophthalmos swelling of both medial recti

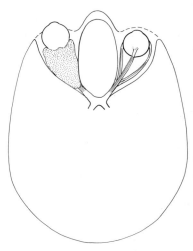

(c) Unilateral exophthalmos due to orbital tumour on left

Fig. 3.8 *Schematic representations of computerised tomographic scans (transverse section of skull through the orbits) indicating the value of this investigation in the differential diagnosis of exophthalmos.*

many of the features may be masked and cardiovascular symptoms often predominate. Hyperthyroidism must always be excluded as a cause of otherwise unexplained weight-loss, proximal myopathy, atrial fibrillation or heart failure. Rarely, hyperthyroidism may also produce an apathetic rather than a hyperkinetic state.

A thyroid crisis or storm is an acceleration of hyperthyroidism which may be precipitated after surgery or stress in a patient whose hyperthyroidism has not been previously recognised or properly treated. It is characterised by pyrexia, cardiac failure and delirium or coma, and requires urgent treatment.

Hyperthyroidism may present in pregnancy and be difficult to distinguish from features of pregnancy *per se*. Maternal immunoglobulins in a mother with Graves' disease may cross the placenta and lead to hyperthyroidism in the neonate. Affected babies have goitre and exophthalmos, pyrexia and tachycardia, and may develop heart failure. Prompt treatment is required but the condition is self-limiting and the immunoglobulins are degraded within a few weeks of birth.

Diagnostic Tests

The clinical diagnosis of hyperthyroidism is confirmed by finding an elevated serum T_4. If the T_4 is normal but thyrotoxicosis is still suspected, then T_3 should be measured. T_3 is often elevated before T_4 in hyperthyroidism (T_3 toxicosis), but other evidence of thyroid autonomy, such as a flat TSH response to TRH or failure of T_3 suppression of radio-iodine uptake, should be sought. Misleading high total T_4 values are found in pregnancy or oral contraceptive therapy due to the effect of oestrogens on TBG capacity and in the rare condition of familial increased TBG. Such patients are clinically euthyroid and the high T_4 can be corrected by direct measurement of TBG or a free thyroxine index, and free T_4 levels are normal. If the diagnosis of hyperthyroidism is still in doubt, or the result of the T_4 or T_3 measurement is at the borderline upper limit of normal, a TRH test should be performed. A normal response to TRH firmly excludes the diagnosis. A flat TSH response to TRH is consistent with hyperthyroidism but may also be found in some patients with ophthalmic Graves' disease who are otherwise euthyroid and in patients with nodular goitres. Radio-iodine uptake studies are rarely necessary except to define a hot nodule and in the diagnosis of a transient thyroiditis.

Management

Before treatments were available, spontaneous remission was known to occur but thyrotoxicosis was often fatal. The choice of treatment is medical, surgical or radio-iodine therapy.

Medical treatment

Antithyroid drugs, such as Carbimazole, its active metabolite Methimazole, or Propylthiouracil, block the synthesis of thyroid hormone. All may produce sensitivity reactions, including skin rash, arthralgia and neutropenia, which rapidly respond to withdrawal of the drug. Sensitivity to one drug does not usually mean sensitivity to another, so if there is a reaction to Carbimazole a patient may be safely put on Propylthiouracil. Very rarely, agranulocytosis may occur and patients should be warned to stop taking the drug if they develop a sore throat or a rash and seek further medical attention immediately. Such reactions usually occur within the first few weeks of treatment if they occur at all. The starting dose of Carbimazole is 30–60 mg daily, and of Propylthiouracil 300–600 mg daily in divided doses. These doses are continued until the patient is euthyroid, usually within a period of six to ten weeks. Biochemical evidence of return to a normal thyroid state is usually evident before it is apparent clinically. Excessive treatment results in a lowered serum T_4 and a rise in TSH. Treatment can be continued by reducing the dose of antithyroid drugs stepwise so as to maintain the patient clinically and biochemically euthyroid. This requires careful supervision at frequent intervals so as to avoid overtreatment or escape due to undertreatment. An alternative approach is to maintain blocking dose of Carbimazole which would, if continued alone, render the patient hypothyroid but, to prevent this, a physiological replacement dose of thyroxine, usually approximately 150 μg daily, is added once the patient is euthyroid – this has the disadvantage of taking extra tablets but avoids the fluctuation of the former regime. Conventionally, antithyroid drug therapy is continued for a year to eighteen months and then withdrawn, but 50–60% of patients will subsequently relapse and alternative therapy should be considered.

β-adrenoceptor blocking drugs such as Propranolol may be used to control the sympathetic effects of hyperthyroidism. They reduce the pulse rate and anxiety and sweating, but weight-loss continues and the patients remain biochemically thyrotoxic, although the drug does reduce conversion of T_4 to T_3. It can be used short-term pending confirmation of the diagnosis or to cover radio-iodine therapy; some centres use it in preparation for surgery but this needs very careful supervision as it only lasts a few hours and omission of a single dose before or after the operation can result in severe hyperthyroidism.

Medical treatment is preferred in children and teenagers or adults not wishing to undergo surgery. Thyrotoxicosis in pregnancy is best treated by as small as possible a dose of Carbimazole alone, since it crosses the placental barrier and can affect the fetus. It is usually possible to control the hyperthyroidism with 5–15 mg daily, and treatment is conventionally stopped two weeks before delivery and renewed after the puerperium if necessary. Carbimazole is excreted in very low doses in the maternal milk, and women are customarily advised not to breastfeed if they are on the drug, but this may not be essential. If the patient cannot be controlled on modest doses of Carbimazole alone, then partial thyroidectomy can be undertaken in mid-pregnancy.

Neonatal hyperthyroidism should be treated with Carbimazole in a dose according to body weight. Potassium iodide drops, Propranolol and digoxin may be necessary in the early acute phase. Carbimazole can be tailed off after about two months.

A thyroid crisis requires emergency treatment with Carbimazole given i.v. or 60–120 mg given by nasogastric tube, and β-blockade. Oral iodine should be given after Carbimazole. Dexamethasone may also be of benefit as it inhibits T_3 production from T_4. Intravenous fluids may be needed but, if cardiac failure occurs, diuretics and digoxin should be given.

The treatment of exophthalmos depends on the severity of the condition. Mild lid retraction and orbital protrusion insufficient to prevent closure of the eyelids requires no treatment. In more severe cases, exposure of the cornea may require protective tarsorraphy to prevent abrasion and ulceration. Ophthalmoplegia leads to diplopia and can be very disturbing as well as disfiguring. Temporarily an eyepatch can relieve some of the distress but, if troublesome ophthalmoplegia persists after correction of the thyroid dysfunction, surgical procedures may be necessary to correct the deformity.

Malignant exophthalmos requires urgent expert treatment to prevent blindness. Several different treatments have been used and include large doses of steroids, cyclosporin, plasmapheresis, surgical decompression of the orbit, and external radiation. It is not easy to make any comparison of the relative merits of each of these procedures because the condition is not readily amenable to controlled clinical trial. Prednisolone in doses of 60 to 100 mg daily can produce a dramatic reduction in papilloedema and improvement in visual acuity, but the side-effects of such large doses of steroids rapidly become apparent. Orbital decompression will lead to rapid reduction of pressure on the eyeball and reduce the protrusion and exposure, but further surgery may be needed later to correct enophthalmos and ocular palsies. The benefits of plasmapheresis are short-lived, and initial claims for its efficacy have not found universal confirmation. External radiation is not usually immediately effective and is used to supplement other treatments.

Surgery

Partial thyroidectomy is appropriate in adults with thyrotoxicosis due to a hot nodule, or a diffuse or multinodular goitre unless the patient is otherwise unsuitable for or does not want surgery. Patients are best treated medically before surgery so that they are euthyroid at the time of operation. Afterwards the antithyroid drugs can be discontinued. It is doubtful whether potassium iodide solution given for a few days before surgery has any beneficial effect on a patient who is already euthyroid on antithyroid drugs. Propranolol alone in the preparation of a patient for surgery is not recommended except in experienced centres with close supervision. There is a slight risk of operative damage to the recurrent laryngeal nerve and of hypoparathyroidism. Postoperative hypocalcaemia may develop within a day or so of operation if there has been damage to the parathyroids, and requires treatment with calcium supplements and, if necessary, vitamin D. Transient hypothyroidism, evidenced by low thyroxine and raised TSH, may occur a few weeks after surgery. It should be observed for a month to see if improvement occurs but should not be allowed to progress to overt hypothyroidism. The vast majority of patients become euthyroid but relapse occurs in about 5% of cases and the cumulative incidence of hypothyroidism may reach 25% or more over ten years.

Radio-iodine therapy

In large doses, ^{131}I destroys the function of thyroid cells and prevents their replication. It is simple to administer and is particularly suitable for the elderly. The therapeutic dose is somewhat arbitrary, 5 mCuries may be sufficient but some patients require up to 15 mCuries to render them euthyroid. Twenty per cent will become hypothyroid within a year, and the cumulative rate of hypothyroidism reaches about 50% after ten years. For this reason, some physicians prefer to give a larger dose in the first place to render the patient hypothyroid and start thyroxine replacement early. Whichever dose is used, it may take several weeks for patients to respond and they may need to be rendered euthyroid in the meantime by the use of antithyroid drugs started just after the radioactive iodine. Carbimazole treatment can be withdrawn after six months to determine the effect of the radio-iodine. An alternative approach is to give a β-adrenoceptor blocking drug such as Propranolol until the patient becomes euthyroid. This allows the effect of the ^{131}I on thyroid function to be monitored. There is no evidence that radio-iodine induces cancer or leukaemia but in the UK it has been conventional not to give therapeutic doses of radio-iodine to women in their reproductive years. Radio-iodine therapy or surgical excision are equally effective treatments for hot nodules.

Whichever form of treatment is chosen for hyperthyroidism, long-term follow-up is essential to detect relapse or the development of hypothyroidism.

HYPOTHYROIDISM

Hypothyroidism is due to low circulating thyroid hormone levels. Iodine deficiency is the major cause worldwide of primary hypothyroidism in children and adults. Apart from this, hypothyroidism in children is rare but may be due to dyshormonogenesis (i.e. where one of the enzymes responsible for the synthesis of thyroid hormones is defective, Fig. 3.3). In adults it is usually due to autoimmune processes and affects approximately 1% of women, with an incidence of between 1 and 2 cases per 1000 women per year. Up to a third of cases may be due to previous destructive therapy to the thyroid by radio-iodine or surgery. It is most common in the fifth and sixth decades and affects women about ten times more commonly than men. Hypothyroidism may also be *secondary* to pituitary tumours or hypothalamic disorders (e.g. craniopharyngioma). Transient hypothyroidism may occur with acute thyroiditis or overtreatment with antithyroid drugs.

Histological examination of the thyroid in patients with autoimmune thyroiditis (Hashimoto's disease) usually shows diffuse lymphocytic infiltration with associated obliteration of the thyroid follicles and varying amounts of fibrosis. Some epithelial cells may remain and are particularly prominent, with oxyphilic staining of the cytoplasm. These are called Askanazy cells and are pathognomonic of the disease.

Clinical Features

Hypothyroidism is insidious and the symptoms and signs of physical and mental slowing are non-specific. Gross hypothyroidism may not be recognised until it has been present for many months or even years. The patient may attribute the condition to ageing, but the physician must be alert to the possibility of the diagnosis, particularly if there has been previous treatment for thyrotoxicosis, or in the elderly with unexplained lethargy, depression or mental confusion. Other symptoms include increased sensitivity to cold, constipation, weight-gain, intermittent claudication and stiffness of the fingers or other joints.

In overt hypothyroidism, the patient may be deaf and the voice gruff. The face is puffy in appearance, with periorbital oedema, the skin is cold and thickened (myxoedema), and the hair coarse and brittle. Cardiovascular features include bradycardia, cardiomegaly and pericardial effusion. Effusions may also develop in the pleural, peritoneal or other body cavities. The relaxation phase of the tendon reflexes is prolonged in severe hypothyroidism but is often normal in less advanced disease. Other neurological features include carpal tunnel syndrome, myotonia and myopathy. Muscle and joint stiffness may mimic polymyalgia rheumatica. A mild anaemia, which is usually normochromic and normocytic but may be macrocytic, is commonly present. The thyroid is frequently not palpable.

Severely hypothyroid patients may present in coma with hypothermia which may be difficult to distinguish from other causes of hypothermia and the diagnosis should be considered in any elderly patient found at home neglected and brought into hospital in a stupor or coma, with or without hypothermia. It constitutes a medical emergency and carries a high mortality.

Whilst any or all of the above features may be present in overt myxoedema, lesser degrees of thyroid failure are extremely difficult to recognise and may only be detected biochemically. In hypothyroidism secondary to pituitary or hypothalamic disease, the above clinical features of primary hypothyroidism are seldom evident, and features of other pituitary hormone deficiencies tend to predominate.

Diagnostic Tests

In overt primary hypothyroidism, serum total T_4 is low and serum TSH raised (Fig. 3.6c). Serum T_3 levels are of no diagnostic value as they are frequently in the normal range even when T_4 is low. Misleadingly low T_4 values are found in hypoproteinaemic states of whatever cause, e.g. nephrotic syndrome or liver failure, familial TBG deficiency or alteration of TBG binding due to competition from drugs such as phenytoin or anabolic steroids. Severe acute or chronic non-thyroid illness results in increased conversion of T_4 to the inactive metabolite, reverse T_3, and T_4 and FTI may be misleadingly low. In all these circumstances, a normal TSH value excludes the diagnosis of primary hypothyroidism. In hypothyroidism secondary to pituitary disease, T_4 values and FTI are low and there is no TSH response to TRH (Fig. 3.6d), but with lesser degrees of pituitary impairment the pattern of TSH response to TRH is variable. In hypothalamic disease, TSH response to TRH is typically delayed (Fig. 3.6e). Rarely, a patient with primary hypothyroidism is found to have an enlarged pituitary fossa on x-ray due to a feedback tumour resulting from prolonged hypertrophy of pituitary thyrotrophs. The high TSH level will distinguish the primary cause from hypothyroidism secondary to pituitary disease.

In primary hypothyroidism, the ECG may reveal bradycardia, low voltage complexes, ST segment depression and T wave inversion, but such changes are not invariably present and are not specific.

Treatment

Patients without cardiovascular complications should be given synthetic thyroxine in an initial dose of 50 μg daily, increased every two weeks until a maintenance dose, usually 150 μg daily, is achieved when T_4 and TSH levels should be within the normal range. In the elderly, or if ischaemic heart disease is present, thyroxine replacement should be more cautious, starting with 25 μg daily and increased every two to four weeks in 25 μg steps until the maintenance dose is achieved. If there is an exacerbation of angina, the dose of thyroxine should be reduced and a β-blocking drug introduced. If there is no further angina, gradual 25 μg increments may be reintroduced until the optimum dose is achieved. An alternative approach is to give low doses of tri-iodothyronine (5 μg 8-hourly). This can be increased more rapidly than thyroxine and, if angina develops, has the advantage that its half-life is shorter that T_4. β-blocking drugs should be avoided in patients who have pericardial effusions when diuretics may also be necessary.

The treatment of myxoedema coma is controversial and empirical. It constitutes a medical emergency and is not amenable to controlled clinical trials. Some authors advise administration of a large intravenous bolus of thyroxine. The present author favours the use of intramuscular T_3 in 10 μg doses, twice daily initially, gradually increasing to 20 μg three times a day. If parenteral T_3 is not available, then the oral preparation can be given via a nasogastric tube (2.5–5.0 μg 8-hourly increasing after 48 hrs to 10 μg 8-hourly). Intramuscular hydrocortisone is also given to counteract any impaired cortisol response to stress, but this can be withdrawn if plasma cortisol taken prior to treatment is subsequently found to be normal. The patient is wrapped in a space blanket to facilitate correction of hypothermia, and adequate ventilation and oxygenation is maintained, if necessary by assisted ventilation. Once awake, gradual substitution therapy with thyroxine can be commenced.

In hypothyroidism secondary to pituitary disease any coexisting cortisol deficiency should be corrected before thyroxine replacement therapy is initiated on similar lines for primary hypothyroidism, and further treatment directed to the cause of the pituitary dysfunction.

Thyroxine replacement therapy should be continued for life. A certain proportion of patients will be non-compliant and may gradually relapse, which creates a need for regular supervison. An indication that adequate therapy is not being maintained in patients with primary hypothyroidism is a rise in serum TSH.

ASYMPTOMATIC AUTOIMMUNE THYROIDITIS

Circulating thyroid microsomal antibodies may be found in approximately 10% of women and 1% of men who are clinically euthyroid, being most common in postmenopausal women. Gastric parietal cell antibodies show a similar age and sex distribution. Many such women will remain euthyroid for the rest of their lives, but about half will be found to have raised serum TSH levels in the presence of normal T_4, indicating a compensatory increased TSH drive. Overt hypothyroidism will develop at the rate of approximately 5% per annum in such people and may justify prophylactic thyroxine replacement therapy.

CONGENITAL HYPOTHYROIDISM

Maternal iodine deficiency can lead to the development of goitrous hypothyroidism and cretinism in the infant in areas of endemic iodine deficiency. It can be prevented by the prophylactic use of intramuscular injections of iodised oil given to women of reproductive years or very early in pregnancy.

In non iodine-deficient areas, congenital hypothyroidism is usually due to an absent or ectopic thyroid and occurs in 1:3500 births. It may be difficult to detect clinically before the infant is several weeks or even months old. It can be identified biochemically at birth by taking a cord blood sample, or five days later by heel-prick at the time of screening for phenylketonuria. In normal infants, there is a surge of TSH within a few hours of birth which normally subsides within two or three days. Routine screening on day five for persistent elevation of TSH should lead to prompt thyroxine replacement therapy and, hopefully, prevent the impaired physical and mental development which may occur if treatment is delayed. Such screening is now undertaken in almost all European countries and in the US.

GOITRE, NODULES AND CANCER

Goitre, with or without hypothyroidism, is endemic in iodine-deficient countries, and over 20% of the population have visible thyroid swellings. In non-endemic areas, diffuse goitre is commonest in young women. Diffuse goitre declines with age but nodular goitre increases in frequency with age. Goitre is at least four times more common in women than in men and there is no age trend in males (Fig. 3.9).

There is physiological enlargement of the thyroid during puberty and pregnancy. Diffuse goitre is usually found in Graves' disease and a firm enlargement of the thyroid is commonly associated with autoimmune thyroiditis (Hashimoto's thyroiditis). Goitrogens include antithyroid drugs and other agents which interfere with

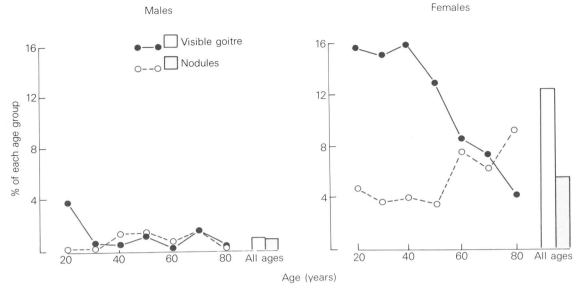

Fig. 3.9 *Age and sex distribution of visible goitre and nodules (based on data from Tunbridge* et al. *(1977)* Clinical Endocrinology 7, 418).

thyroid hormone synthesis or release, e.g. iodine-containing medication, aminoglutethimide and lithium, and certain foodstuffs such as soyabean and cassava. Goitre and hypothyroidism in childhood is rare and may be due to familial dyshormonogenesis. The latter includes enzyme defects in one or more of the various steps in thyroid hormone synthesis and release – iodide trapping, organification, coupling, deiodination and impaired thyroglobulin synthesis (see thyroid hormone formation and Fig. 3.3). Congenital deafness and goitre associated with an organification defect is known as Pendred's syndrome. Whilst the above conditions may account for some cases of benign sporadic goitre, the aetiology is unknown in the majority of cases and may be due to growth-stimulating factors other than TSH. Some immunoglobulins appear to stimulate growth, but not functioning of the gland, and vice versa.

Thyroid cancers are comparatively rare and account for less than 0.5% of all deaths due to malignant disease. Age-specific death rates from thyroid cancer in all ages in the UK are about 5 per million men and about 15 per million women per year. Thyroid cancers are found most frequently in women aged 45–65.

Solitary nodules in the thyroid may be due to papillary or follicular carcinoma, which must be distinguished from benign adenoma, cysts or haematomas. Benign adenomas are common and well encapsulated. Papillary carcinoma is the commonest form of thyroid cancer, the capsule is incomplete and metastases to cervical lymph glands are common and may be more widespread. Follicular carcinomas vary in size and degree of differentiation, and distant metastases are common. Anaplastic carcinomas are large and infiltrate the whole gland and surrounding tissues. Other rarer tumours include medullary carcinomas, (C-cell tumours which secrete calcitonin), and infiltration by lymphoma. Rarely, granulomata of sarcoidosis, tuberculosis or syphilis may be found in the thyroid.

Clinical Features

The patient may complain of a lump in the neck, or the goitre may be noticed incidentally on routine clinical examination. Symptomatic enquiry should be made to assess possible hyper- or hypofunction (see above). The history should always include an enquiry into the patient's medication, particularly cough mixtures containing iodine and other goitrogens. Past history of irradiation of the neck in childhood (this used to be done for lymphadenopathy in the US) raises the possibility of a malignancy. Rarely, a gland may be sufficiently large to cause tracheal compression or involvement of the recurrent laryngeal nerve, presenting with stridor and/or hoarse voice. A painful goitre is uncommon and is usually due to subacute (De Quervain's) thyroiditis but may follow a therapeutic dose of radio-iodine and is very occasionally due to acute suppuration.

The finding of a solitary nodule or history of a rapidly-enlarging gland always requires investigation to exclude a malignancy. A solitary nodule may be cystic or solid, and it is difficult on clinical examination to decide whether it is benign or malignant. Involvement of cervical lymph nodes is highly suggestive of malignancy, but can be found in benign autoimmune thyroiditis. A solitary midline nodule may be due to a thyroglossal cyst.

Anaplastic carcinomas are usually hard, tender, irregular and fixed to surrounding tissues. A woody, hard gland is also found in the rare Riedel's thyroiditis, which may be associated with retroperitoneal fibrosis. Medullary carcinoma may be associated with multiple neuromas in the eyelids, lips and tongue, and evidence for associated hyperparathyroidism and phaeochromocytoma should be sought.

Investigations

Investigations are directed towards determining the level of thyroid function and the cause of the goitre and its effects. Hyperthyroidism and hypothyroidism should be excluded (pp. 55 and 58). In an apparently euthyroid patient, serum thyroxine and TSH may be normal but serum T_3 may be slightly elevated. A flat TSH response to TRH is not uncommon in patients with nodular goitres who are otherwise biochemically euthyroid. The presence of thyroid antibodies indicates an underlying autoimmune process but does not exclude the possibility of coexistent malignant change.

Radio-iodine uptake studies may be helpful in defining the cause of dyshormonogenetic goitre (see above); the main value of isotopes is for scanning to define the size and position of the goitre, particularly if retrosternal, and location of ectopic thyroid tissue and to establish the functional activity of thyroid nodules (Fig. 3.10). An ultrasonic scan may be helpful in defining whether a cold nodule (i.e. inactive on isotope scan) greater than 1 cm in diameter is purely cystic, semisolid or solid, but the diagnosis ultimately depends on biopsy findings.

Fine needle aspiration in skilled hands, together with expert cytology or histology, may obviate the need for time-consuming and expensive scans. Such expertise is not usually available except in specialist centres, and surgical exploration is otherwise advised for all cold nodules.

Management

Benign goitre

The majority of goitres are benign and not associated with disordered thyroid function. The patient requires reassurance to this effect. Hyperthyroidism or hypothyroidism should be treated as appropriate (pp. 55 and 58). The patient with an autonomous nodule who is clinically and biochemically euthyroid may be kept under observation. A proportion will develop hyperthyroidism, often first indicated by a rise in serum T_3, which can be treated with surgery or radio-iodine. Large glands may warrant surgery for cosmetic reasons, but a trial of thyroxine replacement therapy may be justified even in the absence of raised TSH, although shrinkage of the gland will only occur in a small proportion. Pressure symptoms require surgical relief.

Subacute thyroiditis should be treated symptomatically. Pain may be relieved by large doses of Prednisolone, which can be gradually reduced over a few weeks. Transient hyperthyroidism (evidenced by high circulating thyroid hormone levels and a low radio-iodine uptake) in the early phase is usually self-limiting. Transient hypothyroidism may follow but is uncommon. Hypothyroidism may develop in patients with Riedel's thyroiditis, and requires standard replacement therapy. This will not reduce the size of the gland;

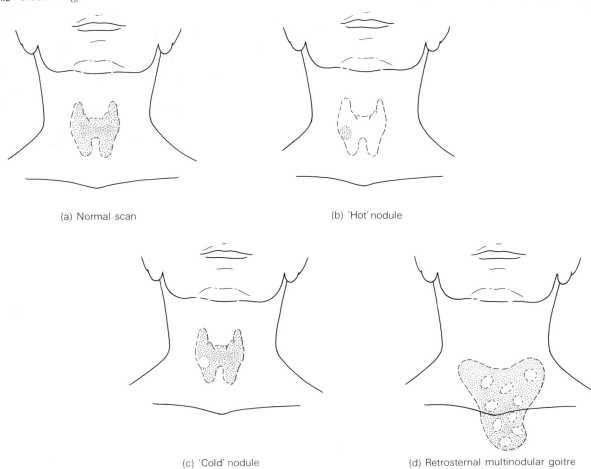

(a) Normal scan

(b) 'Hot' nodule

(c) 'Cold' nodule

(d) Retrosternal multinodular goitre

Fig. 3.10 *Radioiodine scans of the thyroid.*

occasionally surgical relief for pressure symptoms is necessary.

Cold nodules and thyroid malignancy

The vast majority of multinodular goitres are benign but may conceal a malignant growth. If there is rapid growth or cervical lymphadenopathy, then exploration is advised. Apparent single nodules are often found to be multiple at exploration, but a solitary cyst should be excised because there is a high risk of recurrence after simple aspiration and malignant changes are occa-

sionally found in the cyst walls. If a papillary or follicular carcinoma is found, then total thyroidectomy in skilled hands is ideally advisable. If such expertise is not readily available, it is safer to advise partial thyroidectomy and subsequent ablation with a large dose of radio-iodine. The patient then requires maintenance therapy with T_3 sufficient to maintain euthyroidism and to suppress TSH. At intervals T_3 is discontinued for 10 days to allow TSH levels to rise and the patient then given radio-iodine to identify any remaining thyroid tissue or metastatic lesions which will require further thera-peutic doses of radio-iodine. With well-differentiated tumours thyroglobulin can be used as a tumour marker. If this is detectable in the patient who has had the normal thyroid tissue ablated, then it would suggest the presence of residual or recurrent tumour. Prognosis for well-differentiated carcinoma, if detected early, is relatively good, with ten-year survival rates of 50% or more. Anaplastic and other poorly-differentiated tumours have a very poor prognosis. Surgical removal should not be attempted, although occasionally limited surgery is necessary to relieve pressure symptoms. Radio-iodine has no effect, and treatment is with palliative external radiation. Medullary carcinoma should be treated by thyroidectomy and excision of lymph node metastases where possible. Plasma calcitonin levels can be measured to monitor the response to treatment and recurrence of metastases. The patient should be investigated to exclude phaeochromocytoma and parathyroid adenomas prior to thyroid surgery, and first-degree relatives should also be screened for evidence of medullary carcinoma and associated endocrine neoplasia.

4

The Adrenal Glands

The adrenal resembles certain other glands, for example the pituitary, in being composed of two parts which are embryologically, anatomically and, apparently, functionally quite separate. The adrenal cortex is derived from mesoderm and is the source of steroid hormones, while the medulla, which is neuroectodermal, secretes catecholamines and peptides. Although conventional, this view may not be strictly accurate and it is possible that the functions of the cortex and medulla are more interrelated than they at first appear: they share a common blood supply and this would allow steroids from the cortex to modulate medullary function. Even their anatomical relationship is not simple: a cuff of cortical tissue lies invaginated within the medulla, surrounding the central vein and its major branches.

Each gland sits like a tricorn hat, a helmet, on the upper pole of the kidney; the left one being rather longer and thinner. The arterial blood supply comes from three sources: aorta, inferior phrenic and renal arteries (Fig. 4.1). Arterioles form a capsular plexus and the capillaries run centripetally through the outer layers of the cortex. As they pass more centrally they give way to sinusoids which form interconnecting pools and finally drain through the medulla to collect in the tributaries of the central vein. The left adrenal vein drains into the left renal vein while the right drains directly into the inferior vena cava.

The medulla receives a rich nerve supply of preganglionic sympathetic fibres from the coeliac ganglia and their derivatives. The secretory cells of the adrenal medulla are essentially equivalent to postganglionic sympathetic neurones without axons. Instead of releasing their chemical messengers from nerve terminals as 'neurotransmitters', they release them into the blood stream as 'hormones'.

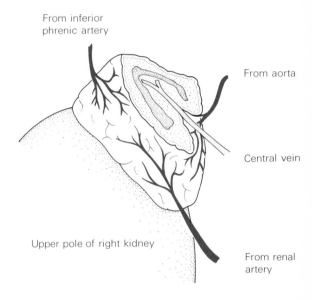

From inferior phrenic artery

From aorta

Central vein

Upper pole of right kidney

From renal artery

Fig. 4.1 *Schematic diagram of right adrenal gland, with the cut surface exposed.*

ADRENAL MEDULLA

Structure

The medulla is composed of a loose network of nerve fibres, ganglia, secretory cells and connective tissue (Fig. 4.2). Through this lattice flows the sinusoidal blood, passing on its way from the cortex to the central vein.

The secretory cells are large and have foamy cytoplasm containing secretory granules. With silver stains these cells stain brown: *chromaffin* tissue.

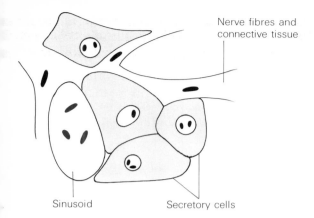

Fig. 4.2 *Structure of the adrenal medulla.*

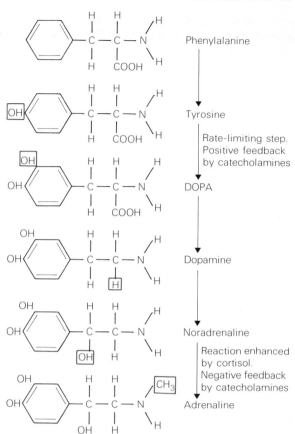

Fig. 4.3 *Synthesis of catecholamines.*

Hormones

The adrenal medulla secretes catecholamlines, dopamine, adrenaline and noradrenaline, in response to impulses received through the preganglionic (cholinergic) sympathetic nerves. There are two populations of secretory cells: those with larger, less dense granules which contain adrenaline, and are commoner; and those with smaller, denser granules containing noradrenaline. There is increasing evidence that both types of cell also produce peptide neurotransmitters such as met-enkephalin, ACTH and somatostatin.

Synthesis of catecholamines

Adrenaline and noradrenaline are derived from the chain conversion of phenylalanine through dopamine (Fig. 4.3). The rate-limiting step is the hydroxylation of tyrosine to DOPA (dihydroxyphenylalanine) by tyrosine hydroxylase, but the speed of this reaction is enhanced by catecholamines themselves. In addition, the conversion of noradrenaline to adrenaline is cortisol-dependent, and this may be a clue to one aspect of the functional interdependence of the two parts of the adrenal gland.

Actions of catecholamines

The actions of catecholamines are mediated via a family of cell-surface receptors, and the relative prevalence of these receptors differs from tissue to tissue. However their actions are so numerous and so widespread that it is difficult to envisage how the release of these hormones from the *adrenal medulla* can be used by the body to induce a specific response. This is especially true if one considers that in most instances adrenaline and noradrenaline are released together from this gland and, as far as is known, some stimuli to their secretion will result also in the secretion of dopamine, and peptide hormones. Either the physiological actions of these hormones are subject to extremely subtle modulation at their many target tissues, or the adrenal medulla may be considered a relatively atavistic and unsubtle gland whose functions have

Table 4.1

Effects of Stimulation of α- and β-adrenoceptors

α-receptors (effects mediated via altered cellular Ca^{++} concentration)
Dilatation of the pupil
Constriction of coronary arteries
Constriction of arterioles in skin, muscle, kidney, gut
Constriction of venules
Contraction of the stomach, bowel, anal sphincter, trigone
Ejaculation
Increased sweating; increased thickness of salivary secretion
Decreased pancreatic endocrine (insulin and glucagon) and exocrine (enzyme) secretion
Increased glycogenolysis (not particularly predominant in man)
Effects in central nervous system: alertness, fear, anxiety

β-receptors (effects mediated via adenyl cyclase)
Increase in cardiac output via increased heart rate, increased contractility, decreased peripheral resistance
Dilatation of coronary, skeletal muscle, renal and pulmonary arteries and arterioles
Relaxation of bronchial smooth muscle
Decreased motility of the gut and bladder detrusor muscle
Increased pancreatic endocrine and exocrine secretion
Increased lipolysis with FFA release
Increased glycogenolysis (predominant pathway in man)

been largely superseded by the postganglionic fibres of the sympathetic nervous system.

Although it is generally accepted that the capacity of the adrenal medulla to release large quantities of catecholamines plays an important role in preparing an animal for 'fight or flight', no harm seems to follow its removal and the real physiological significance of medullary catecholamines, and peptides, remains unknown.

Actions of noradrenaline and adrenaline

The main effects of circulating catecholamines are seen in the cardiovascular system, the central nervous system and in carbohydrate and lipid metabolism. The effects are mediated through the stimulation of the four classes of sympathetic receptor: designated α_1, α_2, β_1 and β_2.

In general, noradrenaline has a predominant effect on α receptors, while adrenaline affects both α and β receptors. Together the two hormones prepare the animal for 'fight or flight' by increasing cardiac output, altering the differential blood supply to tissues (with increased circulation to e.g., skeletal muscle and liver), inducing mental alertness, and releasing nutrients (carbohydrate and free fatty acids) from liver and

Table 4.2

Effect of Certain Drugs on Catecholamine Metabolism

Action	Drug	Clinical value	Undesirable clinical effect
Stimulation of catecholamine release	Nicotine Tyramine Ephedrine Amphetamine	Ephedrine for asthma, nasal congestion Amphetamine for narcolepsy	Addiction (nicotine, amphetamine) tremor, sleeplessness
Decreased catecholamine release (false transmitter)	α-methyldopa α-methylpara-tyrosine (AMPT)	Methyldopa for hypertension	Depression
Decreased release and reuptake	Reserpine Guanethidine Bretylium	Formerly used for hypertension	Depression, diarrhoea
Decreased breakdown	MAO inhibitors	Depression	Hypertension, if any sympathetic stimulant given in addition

Table 4.3

Some Effects of Certain Drugs on Catecholamine Receptors

Action	Drug	Clinical value	Undesirable clinical effect
α_1 stimulant	Phenylephrine	Nasal congestion	Sympathetic stimulation
α_2 stimulant	Clonidine	Hypertension	Rebound hypertension with cessation
α blockade	Phenoxybenzamine	Preparation of phaeochromocytoma	Hypotension
	Prazosin	Hypertension, heart failure	Hypotension
β_1 stimulant	Isoprenaline Dopamine Dobutamine Theophylline	Low cardiac output, cardiogenic shock Asthma	Tremor
β_2 stimulant	Salbutamol Theophylline	Asthma	Tremor
β_1 blockade	e.g. Metoprolol	Hypertension, ischaemic heart disease	Decreased peripheral circulation, heart block
β blockade	e.g. Propranolol	Hypertension	Depression, bronchospasm, cold hands and feet
Dopamine stimulant	Bromocriptine	Hyperprolactinaemia	Nausea, postural hypotension
Dopamine blockade	Haloperidol	Psychosis, mania	Hyperprolactinaemia

muscle. Some of the detailed effects of stimulation of α and β receptors are given in Table 4.1. Effects of certain drugs on catecholamine metabolism and catecholamine receptors are given in Tables 4.2 and 4.3.

Actions of dopamine

Dopamine has specific receptors but interacts also with β adrenergic receptors. Infusion in man leads to increased cardiac output, but with specific increase in renal perfusion. It is for this reason that dopamine and related drugs have been widely used in the treatment of cardiogenic shock. However, the physiological significance of circulating dopamine is unknown.

Actions of peptide hormones of the adrenal medulla

Enkephalins and somatostatin have specific receptors in many tissues but the physiological significance of their release, as well as that of other peptides, from the adrenal medulla is unknown. However, nicotine (and amphetamine) release the opioid (morphine-like) peptide, met-enkephalin from the adrenal medulla, and it is tempting to speculate that this action may underlie the addictive effect of smoking. However, it is not thought that circulating opioid peptides cross the blood–brain barrier, and the evidence for such a mechanism is slight.

Metabolic clearance of catecholamines

There are three main pathways of catecholamine clearance:

i. Excretion unchanged into the urine (very small amounts).
ii. Uptake by liver, muscle and sympathetic nerve terminals.
iii. Enzymatic breakdown by monoamine oxidase (MAO) and catechol-O-methyltransferase (COMT) to metanephrines, normetanephrines and VMA (Fig. 4.4).

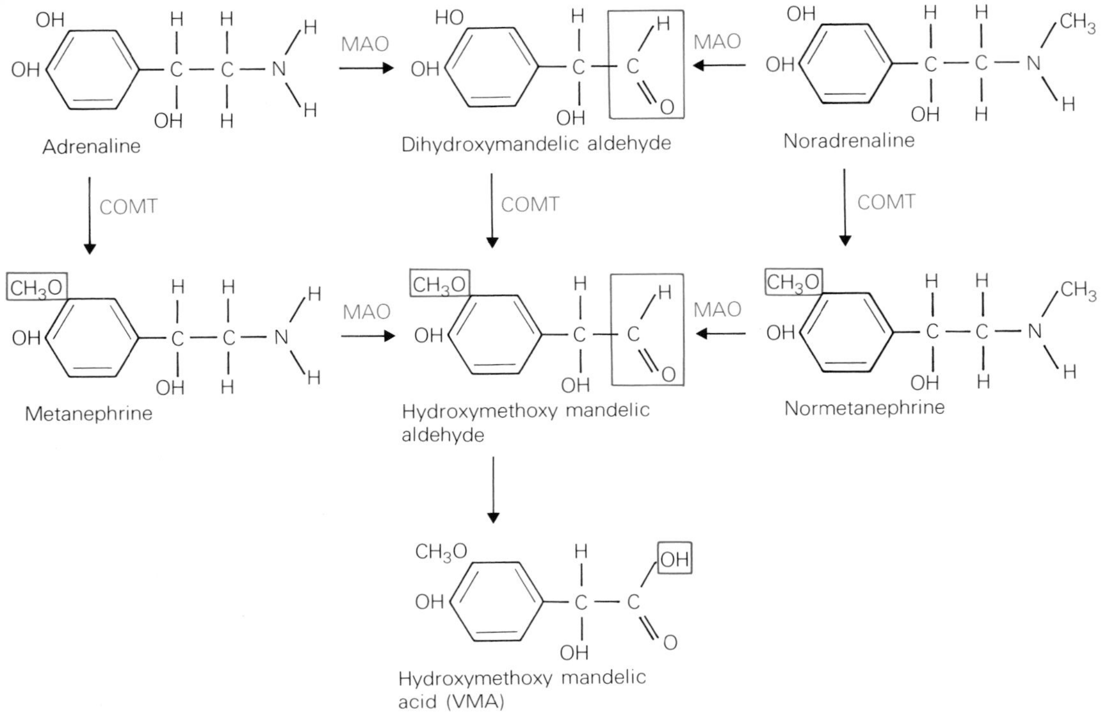

Fig. 4.4 *Metabolic breakdown of catecholamines.*

Measurement of plasma and urinary catecholamines

Hitherto it has always been difficult to measure catecholamines in blood but, now that plasma methods have become more sensitive and more robust, it is possible that plasma assays will replace the conventional 24-hour urine measurement.

Plasma: Although adrenaline-secreting cells outnumber catecholamine-secreting cells in the adrenal medulla, the concentration of adrenaline in blood (approximately 0.15 nmol/l) is only about one-tenth that of noradrenaline. Since the half-life of each is similar (approximately 2 mins), this reflects the derivation of plasma noradrenaline from other sources – notably postganglionic sympathetic nerve terminals. However,

the enzyme necessary for the formation of adrenaline from noradrenaline (phenylethanolamine-N-methyl transferase) occurs only in the adrenal medulla and brain, and is not found elsewhere in the autonomic nervous system. Following adrenalectomy, plasma adrenaline levels fall to very low levels, whereas those of noradrenaline, dopamine and met-enkephalin do not fall so much, if at all.

Urine: The urine may be analysed for catecholamines (total, including conjugated, or free), metanephrines or normetanephrines (the major excretory products of adrenaline and noradrenaline), vanillyl mandelic acid (VMA, HMMA) or homovanillic acid (HVA, the major excretory product of dopamine). Very small amounts of the catecholamines are excreted unchanged.

Table 4.4

Some Factors that Interfere with Measurement of Catecholamine Excretory Products

a. *Biological*
Stress, illness and physical exertion.
Diet: coffee, bananas, some nuts but NOT vanilla. Tyrosine-containing foods
  (e.g. cheese) may affect plasma assays.
Drugs: MAO inhibitors, disulfiram (Antabuse). β-blocking drugs more
  likely to affect plasma assays than urinary ones.

b. *Artefactual*
Interference with the assay procedure: dependent on method employed.
  Methyldopa, labetalol, tetracycline, chlorpromazine.

Normally, about 35% is excreted in the form of VMA, but in some phaeochromocytomas the percentage may be much smaller, and for clinical purposes it is preferable to assay catecholamines and/or metanephrines. Many factors may interfere with plasma and urinary assays and the advice of the local Department of Chemical Pathology should always be sought before samples are collected. The interference may be biological (foodstuffs, effects of stress or drugs on the body) or artefactual (see Table 4.4). It should be noted that – despite oft-quoted dogma – ingestion of vanilla has no effect on catecholamine excretory products, and the ingestion of foods such as bananas has to be simian to be significant.

Diseases of the Adrenal Medulla

Early animal experiments showed that bilateral removal of the adrenal medulla could be performed without permanent ill-effect and, similarly, there are no recognised clinical syndromes resulting from medullary hypofunction. Diseases of the adrenal medulla are solely those of tumour formation, with or without associated endocrine overactivity. There are several types of tumour, and all are rare:

1. Tumour of neuroblasts – neuroblastoma.
2. Tumour of ganglion cells – ganglioneuroma.
3. Tumour of chromaffin cells – phaeochromocytoma.

Neuroblastoma

With an annual incidence in the UK of approximately 80, this is one of the commonest childhood tumours; it tends to be highly malignant. More than 90% are endocrinologically active but, because of its malignancy, many children present with metastases rather than with the effects of excessive catecholamine secretion (in contrast to phaeochromocytoma, see below). Treatment of neuroblastoma is by excision, if possible, followed by radiotherapy and/or chemotherapy.

Ganglioneuroma

Ganglioneuromas are much less common than neuroblastomas, and tend to occur in older children and young adults. They may also secrete catecholamines, and tend to be more benign in their behaviour.

Phaeochromocytoma

The overall annual incidence of phaeochromocytoma is of the same order as neuroblastoma, but it is a tumour of adults and as such is relatively uncommon. It is also a rare cause of hypertension, and it is doubtful if the incidence justifies the cost and inconvenience of routine screening of urinary catecholamines in all patients with high blood pressure.

The effects of a hormonally-active phaeochromocytoma are those of excessive catecholamine secretion: hypertension (sustained or paroxysmal), anxiety, palpi-

CASE HISTORY

A 52 year old housewife was referred to hospital with mild diabetes. She had been known to have hypertension for 6 years and had grade III hypertensive retinopathy. When she complained of unexplained panic attacks, urinary catecholamines were measured:

Free catecholamines 2230 and 2450 nmol/day
(Normal 0–680)

The presence of a left adrenal tumour was confirmed on CT scan. After treatment with propanolol and phenoxybenzamine the tumour was removed

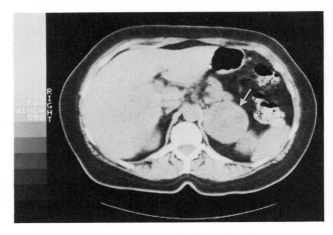

CT scan of the abdomen showing
left adrenal tumour

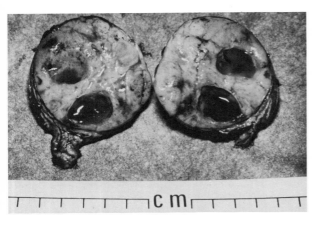

Cut surface of the tumour
after removal

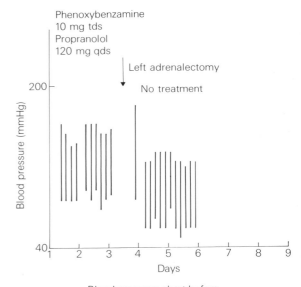

Blood pressure chart before
and after left adrenalectomy

Fig. 4.5 *Phaeochromocytoma (see text).*

tations, pallor, sweating and glucose intolerance (Fig. 4.5). The tumours are usually small and rarely present with an obvious mass. About 10% are multiple (including the other adrenal and sites anywhere in the thoracic and abdominal sympathetic chain) and only about 10% behave in a malignant fashion. There is increasing evidence that phaeochromocytomas may secrete somatostatin and methionine-enkephalin in addition to catecholamines, but the clinical consequences of this are not clear. Occasionally phaeochromocytomas are the source of ectopic ACTH secretion and the patient may present with Cushing's syndrome.

Mixed syndromes

Von Recklinghausen's disease: A tendency to single or multiple phaeochromocytomas is associated with familial neurofibromatosis, von Recklinghausen's disease. These patients also have a predisposition to tumours of other neuroectodermal derivatives, e.g. glioma, orbital tumours, medullary carcinoma of the thyroid.

Multiple endocrine adenomatosis: Occasionally, the presence of an endocrinologically-active tumour of the adrenal medulla may accompany tumours of other endocrine glands: pituitary, parathyroid, pancreas and medullary carcinoma of the thyroid.

Mixed hormone-secreting phaeochromocytomas: Tumours have been described which secrete both catecholamines and ACTH.

Diagnosis of phaeochromocytoma

Diagnosis rests on confirmation of clinical suspicion by demonstrating, 1, elevation of plasma catecholamines or of urinary catecholamines, metanephrines or VMA and, 2, a tumour. The tumour may be shown by plain abdominal x-ray, intravenous urography or computerised tomography of the abdomen. Occasionally it can only be localised by selective venous sampling for catecholamines. The presence of the tumour can be confirmed also by angiography but this, like selective venous sampling, should only be undertaken after careful preparation (see *Dangers,* below). Scintigraphy using radioactively labelled meta-iodo-benzylguanidine is an alternative method for localising benign or malignant phaeochromocytomas.

Treatment of phaeochromocytoma

Phaeochromocytomas are best treated by excision but if for any reason complete removal is not possible, the effects of excessive catecholamine secretion can be controlled by treatment with a combination of α- and β-adrenoceptor blocking drugs: e.g. phenoxybenza-

mine and propranolol. An alternative is α-methylpara-tyrosine (AMPT), which inhibits the conversion of tyrosine to DOPA.

Dangers of investigation and treatment

The main risk is of inducing the release of large quantities of catecholamines, with an accompanying potentially catastrophic rise in blood pressure. For this reason, maximal α- and β-blockade should always be achieved prior to any angiography, selective venous sampling, laparotomy or other manipulation. During surgery sodium nitroprusside is the drug of choice for the control of rapid increases in blood pressure. After complete removal of a phaeochromocytoma there is the additional danger of immediate postoperative hypotensive collapse because patients with chronic vasoconstriction have reduced blood volume. However, the risk of postoperative hypotension is much reduced by adequate preparation with adrenoceptor blocking drugs.

ADRENAL CORTEX

'The physiology of the adrenal glands must be of the greatest importance, but our knowledge of it is amazingly limited. The most important and certain fact is that removal or destruction of both adrenals is invariably followed by death. It is the loss of the cortex, not the medulla, which proves fatal.' (William Boyd. *Textbook of Pathology,* 3rd Edn., 1938.)

Many major discoveries have been made about the physiology of the adrenal cortex since this was written, but the fundamental truth remains: deprivation of adrenocortical hormones is rapidly fatal. It is for this reason that all practising clinicians need to be able to recognise, diagnose accurately and treat adrenocortical failure, even though they may choose to leave the complexities of other adrenal diseases to specialists in the field.

Structure

The adrenal cortex is mesodermal in origin and is comprised of cells which are capable of producing

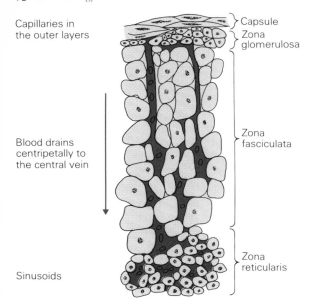

Capillaries in
the outer layers

Blood drains
centripetally to
the central vein

Sinusoids

Capsule
Zona
glomerulosa

Zona
fasciculata

Zona
reticularis

Fig. 4.6 *Structure of the adrenal cortex.*

steroid hormones from cholesterol. The cortex is divided into three zones (Fig. 4.6) and each zone is the source of a different group of steroids, with different overall function.

The outer layer, the *zona glomerulosa,* is composed of small clusters of compact cells (Latin: *glomerulus,* small rounded cluster) which lie beneath the capsule and are the source of aldosterone, the major mineralocorticoid. The cells in the middle layer, the *zona fasciculata,* are larger and are arranged in radiating cords (Latin: *fasciculus,* a small bundle). The abundant cytoplasm of the zona fasciculata appears foamy under the light microscope and is largely composed of storage lipid. The zona fasciculata is the main source of the glucocorticoids, notably cortisol. The innermost layer, the *zona reticularis,* is composed of smaller cells arranged in a loosely reticular pattern and is the main source of adrenal sex steroids.

Hormones

The basic ring structure of these adrenocortical steroids is shown in Fig. 4.7. There are three main groups based

on their principal metabolic effects: *mineralocorticoids* (e.g. aldosterone, deoxycorticosterone), *glucocorticoids* (e.g. cortisol, corticosterone) and *sex steroids* (predominantly androgens). The zona glomerulosa also contains somatostatin, which may play a local or paracrine role in the control of aldosterone secretion.

Mineralocorticoids

The main pathways involved in the synthesis of adrenal steroids are shown in Fig. 4.8. The mineralocorticoids have 21 carbon atoms (C21 steroids). Cortisol and its precursors are also C21 steroids but have an OH group as well as the side-chain on the 17 position (17-hydroxy-

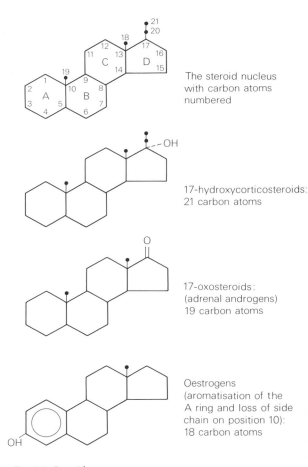

The steroid nucleus with carbon atoms numbered

17-hydroxycorticosteroids: 21 carbon atoms

17-oxosteroids: (adrenal androgens) 19 carbon atoms

Oestrogens (aromatisation of the A ring and loss of side chain on position 10): 18 carbon atoms

Fig. 4.7 *Steroid structure.*

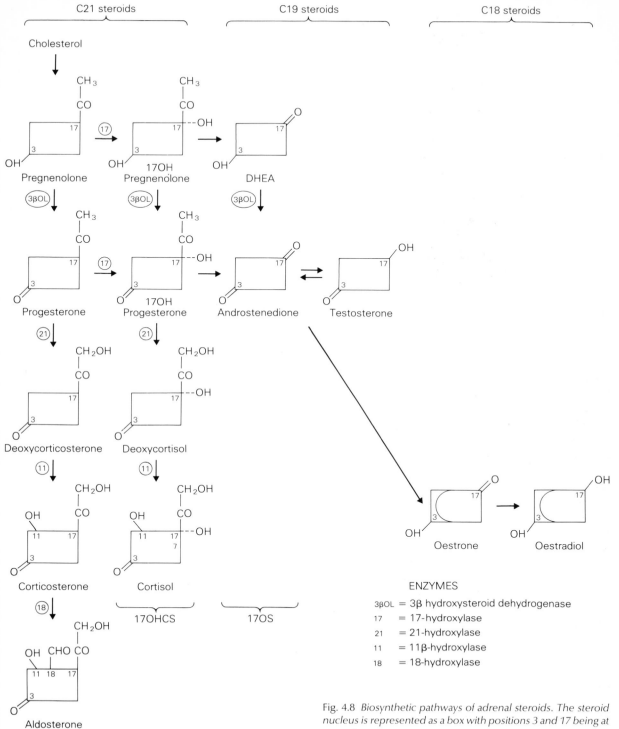

Fig. 4.8 *Biosynthetic pathways of adrenal steroids. The steroid nucleus is represented as a box with positions 3 and 17 being at opposite corners.*

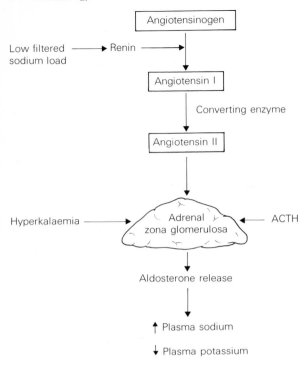

Fig. 4.9 *Control of aldosterone secretion.*

of potassium and hydrogen. They are thus one of many factors concerned with the regulation of sodium, water and acid-base balance. Glucocorticoids have some sodium-retaining action, although the main mineralocorticoid is aldosterone. Aldosterone release appears to be under two main controls: 1. renin-dependent, and 2. renin-independent (see Fig. 4.9).

The renin-dependent system responds to a falling filtered load of sodium in the renal glomerulus or a reduction in pressure in the afferent glomerular arteriole. Renin is released from the juxtaglomerular apparatus and catalyses the conversion of blood-borne angiotensinogen to angiotensin I. Angiotensin converting enzyme (present in the lung and vascular endothelium) then converts the decapeptide angiotensin I into the octapeptide angiotensin II which, in turn, induces the secretion of aldosterone. However, aldosterone release may also be directly stimulated by hyperkalaemia and by adrenocorticotrophic hormone (ACTH) independent of renin.

Glucocorticoids

The actions of glucocorticoids are complex but the main ones are listed in Table 4.5. They are synthesised and released in response to ACTH secretion by the pituitary and ACTH itself is under three main regulatory systems: stress, negative feedback by glucocorticoids and inherent circadian rhythmicity with low levels at midnight and high levels in the morning. The major glucocorticoid cortisol circulates principally bound to an α-globulin, cortisol binding globulin (CBG).

corticosteroids). The adrenal androgens have neither the OH group nor the side-chain on position 17 but have a ketone group in its place (17-oxosteroids).

Mineralocorticoids act on the distal convoluted tubule of the kidney to conserve sodium at the expense

Table 4.5

Main Actions of Glucocorticoids

1. Maintain life.
2. Carbohydrate metabolism: raise blood glucose through gluconeogenesis, but also stimulate glycogenolysis.
3. Protein metabolism: increased breakdown with overall negative nitrogen balance.
4. Suppression of inflammatory response.
5. Increase in neutrophils with decrease in eosinophils.
6. Minor effect on sodium retention and potassium excretion.
7. Suppression of ACTH secretion.
8. Necessary for the normal excretion of a water load.

Sex steroids

Although small amounts of testosterone are secreted by the adrenal, the main androgens produced are weak ones: dehydroepiandrosterone (DHEA) and androstenedione. Conversion of androgens (19 carbon atoms) to oestrogens (18 carbon atoms) is achieved by the aromatisation of the A-ring and removal of the small side chain on C10 (Figs. 4.7 and 4.8). ACTH is probably the main factor controlling sex steroid synthesis and release, although others have been suggested.

Metabolic Clearance of Corticosteroids

Steroids are inactivated by reduction, conjugation and sulphation, and only a small percentage is excreted unchanged. Several different assays are available for the measurement of urinary steroids but the ones most commonly used are:

i. Urine free cortisol – measures unchanged cortisol.
ii. 11-OH corticosteroids – measures all steroids (including cortisol) with an OH group on C11.
iii. 17-OH corticosteroids – measures cortisol and its 17–OH precursors.
iv. 17-oxosteroids – measures the weak adrenal androgens, DHEA and androstenedione.

Effects of Glucocorticoid and Mineralocorticoid Deficiency

Chronic deficiency of glucocorticoids induces weakness, lassitude and weight loss associated with gastrointestinal upset and poor resistance to infection. The low level of cortisol activates the negative feedback control system and results in high levels of ACTH and related peptides which then produce skin pigmentation. Deficiency of mineralocorticoids leads to increased sodium and water-loss with falling blood volume, and consequent postural hypotension and faintness on standing. The plasma potassium concentration rises and sodium falls. Acute glucocorticoid and mineralocorticoid deficiency will result from bilateral adrenalectomy or, spontaneously, from adrenal infarction (such as is classically described in overwhelming meningococcal septicaemia: Waterhouse–Friderickson syndrome – even though it is now thought that hypoadrenalism actually plays little part in the high mortality of this condition). An acute crisis may also be precipitated by intercurrent stress in a patient with chronic adrenocortical insufficiency (Addisonian crisis) and is characterised by hypotensive collapse, fever, hypoglycaemia, abdominal pain and, if untreated, confusion, convulsions and death.

Effects of Adrenal Sex Steroid Deficiency

Provided that the gonads are functioning, adrenal sex steroid deficiency is without clinical effect. However, if there is associated gonadal failure (for instance, in those with a pituitary tumour who have combined ACTH and gonadotrophin deficiency) axillary, pubic and facial hair are lost.

Effects of Glucocorticoid Excess

The effect of excessive cortisol secretion is to produce Cushing's syndrome (Fig 4.10). Fat accumulates around the abdomen, head and neck, while it is lost from the arms and legs. Blood sugar rises and the patient has a tendency to diabetes mellitus. The effect of cortisol in promoting protein catabolism (with increased gluconeogenesis) results in negative nitrogen balance with muscle wasting and weakness. There is thinning of the skin and subcutaneous tissues with bruising and livid abdominal striae, and thinning of the bones with a marked tendency to osteoporotic collapse of the thoracic and lumbar spine, and to asymptomatic rib fractures. The weak mineralocorticoid action of cortisol leads to sodium retention, hypertension and, sometimes, hypokalaemia. Patients also have ankle swelling, usually attributed to the mineralocorticoid effect of cortisol. Depression and other psychiatric disturbances are common, while associated hypersecretion of adrenal androgens from the overactive adrenal cortex leads in women to hirsutism, acne and menstrual disturbance.

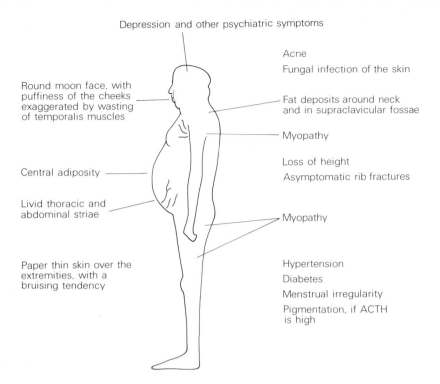

Depression and other psychiatric symptoms

Round moon face, with puffiness of the cheeks exaggerated by wasting of temporalis muscles

Central adiposity

Livid thoracic and abdominal striae

Paper thin skin over the extremities, with a bruising tendency

Acne
Fungal infection of the skin

Fat deposits around neck and in supraclavicular fossae

Myopathy

Loss of height
Asymptomatic rib fractures

Myopathy

Hypertension
Diabetes
Menstrual irregularity
Pigmentation, if ACTH is high

Fig. 4.10 *Clinical features of Cushing's syndrome.*

Effects of Mineralocorticoid Excess

Primary hypersecretion of aldosterone (Conn's syndrome) leads to marked sodium retention with hypertension and hypokalaemic alkalosis. Interestingly, ankle swelling is not a feature of the sodium retention of Conn's. Hyperaldosteronism may also result as part of the compensation for low blood volume in cirrhosis, nephrotic syndrome and congestive heart failure (secondary hyperaldosteronism). In these circumstances the patient is not hypertensive but has a tendency to hypokalaemia.

Effects of Sex Steroid Excess

Adrenal tumours which secrete oestrogens are ex-

tremely rare, but will cause feminisation (gynaecomastia and altered body-fat distribution) in men. More commonly adrenal tumours will result in increased androgen secretion. In the adult male these androgens have no obvious effect, but in women excessive androgens cause hirsutism with or without temporal recession of head hair, acne or menstrual irregularity. When secreted in greater excess, androgens cause *virilisation* with clitoromegaly, increased muscle bulk and deepening voice. In young children the effect of androgens is to produce a temporary stimulation of growth, muscle bulk and strength, followed by early epiphyseal fusion and stunting of final height (see *Congenital Adrenal Hyperplasia*, below).

DISEASES OF THE ADRENAL CORTEX

Addison's Disease: Primary Adrenocortical Failure

Aetiology

Addison's disease may occur at any age and is usually the result of autoimmune or idiopathic atrophy, with lymphocytic infiltration of the affected, wasted glands. In approximately 50% of cases it is possible to identify adrenal autoantibodies which are presumed to be responsible for the atrophy. Tuberculosis is now an uncommon cause of Addison's disease but, before the Second World War, tuberculous cases outnumbered autoimmune ones by 10:1. Rare causes are haemochromatosis and other infiltrations, haemorrhage and bilateral metastatic deposits.

Clinical signs and symptoms

The patient presents with the symptoms and signs of chronic glucocorticoid and mineralocorticoid deficiency, but not infrequently the diagnosis is first made when the patient is in Addisonian crisis. In such cases abdominal pain, fever and hypotensive collapse may simulate a surgical emergency. However, the correct diagnosis will be suggested by the presence of pigmentation of the skin and mucous membranes, which is caused by very high circulating levels of ACTH and related pituitary peptides. Pigmentation may produce a diffuse duskiness of the whole body but affects especially nipples, scrotum and labia, knuckles, axillary creases, pressure areas, recent scars, palmar creases, lips and buccal mucosa. Sometimes longitudinal streaks of pigment are seen beneath the finger nails.

Diagnosis of Addison's disease

Examination of the blood will usually reveal hyponatraemia with hyperkalaemia and evidence of haemoconcentration. Eosinophilia may be noted, and a random urine sample will contain an inappropriately high sodium concentration. Plasma cortisol will be normal or frankly low, but the most sensitive diagnostic assay is *plasma ACTH,* since levels are nearly always grossly elevated in an attempt to drive the failing glands. However, the ACTH assay is time-consuming and expensive, and requires a high degree of technical expertise, and most clinicians rely on an ACTH stimulation test. A synthetic fragment of ACTH (tetracosactrin, Synacthen) comprising the first 24 amino acids is usually used, and the object of the test is to demonstrate failure of the cortisol rise which normally follows an intramuscular or intravenous injection of 250 μg. Subsidiary investigations include assay of adrenal antibodies and x-ray of the adrenal areas for evidence of tuberculous calcification.

Treatment of Addisonian crisis

The intravenous administration of saline is of greater immediate importance than the administration of hydrocortisone, although in practice both are always given together. Most of the symptoms at presentation

---

Table 4.6

Emergency Treatment of Hypoadrenalism (Addisonian Crisis)

1. Bed rest.
2. Encourage oral fluids if patient able to tolerate them.
3. Intravenous infusion of 0.9% NaCl. 1 l in first hour, 500 ml in second, third and fourth hours, more slowly thereafter. Speed of infusion should be reduced in the elderly and those with cardiovascular disease.
   Calculate total saline deficiency from patient's overall weight loss (1 kg loss roughly equivalent to 1 l saline deficiency).
4. Parenteral hydrocortisone. 50–100 mg IV each 6 hours until infusion discontinued. Continue with reducing doses of oral hydrocortisone.

can be related to the low blood volume, and the administration of hydrocortisone alone will not correct this quickly. None the less any intravenous infusion must be undertaken with caution because it is possible to precipitate pulmonary oedema, even in the young. Treatment of Addisonian crisis is usually given before the results of cortisol measurement are available (see Table 4.6).

Maintenance treatment

Glucocorticoid replacement must be given, either as hydrocortisone (usual dose 20 mg on waking and 10 mg at tea time) or, less commonly, as cortisone acetate (25 mg and 12.5 mg), prednisolone (5 mg and 2.5 mg) or dexamethasone (0.5 mg and 0.25 mg). Aldosterone deficiency can be corrected with the synthetic mineralocorticoid, fludrocortisone (usually 0.05 or 0.1 mg daily). It is not necessary to replace sex steroid deficiency, or catecholamines which may have been lost if the medulla is destroyed coincidentally, e.g. in tuberculous and metastatic cases. During intercurrent illness the patient should be warned to double the hydrocortisone (but not the fludrocortisone) dose and, if he is unable to take tablets because of sickness, he should call his doctor immediately as parenteral hydrocortisone will be required.

Secondary adrenocortical failure

When adrenal atrophy occurs as the result of ACTH deficiency, it is not necessary to give fludrocortisone because the zona glomerulosa is preserved and aldosterone secretion is normal.

Schmidt's syndrome

Patients with autoimmune Addison's disease have a tendency to other autoimmune glandular diseases, especially diabetes, myxoedema and thyrotoxicosis. Such pluriglandular disease appears to be particularly associated with HLA subtype B8 DRW3, and is often referred to as Schmidt's syndrome (even though the condition which Schmidt originally described was lymphocytic infiltration of the thyroid in patients dying with Addison's disease in the early part of this century). Care needs to be exercised in making the diagnosis of myxoedema in previously untreated Addison's disease

because hypoadrenalism itself may cause a low serum thyroxine level with a rise in TSH. These changes would normally be very suggestive of primary thyroid failure, but they correct over a period of months when the Addison's disease is treated.

Cushing's Syndrome

Aetiology

There are four main causes of the increased cortisol secretion which is the essential feature of Cushing's syndrome:

1. Drugs: ACTH or steroid treatment.
2. Increased pituitary secretion of ACTH (Cushing's *disease*).
3. Excessive ACTH from a non-pituitary source (ectopic ACTH syndrome).
4. Adrenal adenoma or carcinoma.

To these may be added a fifth: Alcohol-induced pseudo-Cushing's syndrome (see below).

Diagnosis

All patients suspected of having Cushing's syndrome should be assessed and managed by specialist units. The diagnosis rests on the demonstration of sustained elevation of cortisol secretion: raised plasma cortisol at midnight (this is the *only* indication for a midnight cortisol sample), and elevated 24-hour urinary cortisol, 11-OHCS or 17-OHCS. In addition, there is resistance to suppression with dexamethasone: this synthetic glucocorticoid normally causes prompt suppression of plasma cortisol, but in Cushing's syndrome, the negative feedback mechanism is impaired. The stress response of ACTH and cortisol is also impaired, and in Cushing's syndrome there is no cortisol response to insulin hypoglycaemia (see Table 4.7).

Differential diagnosis

a. Adrenal tumour (adenoma and carcinoma)

Adrenal tumours (usually adenomas) account for only 10% of cases in adults, but in children *carcinoma* of the adrenal is the commonest cause of Cushing's syndrome. The tumour may be palpable or it may be

Table 4.7

Diagnosis of Cushing's Syndrome

1. Clinical.
2. Biochemical.
   a. Elevated 24-hour urine steroid excretion (free cortisol or 11-OHCS).
   b. Loss of circadian rhythm of plasma cortisol.
   c. Resistance to suppression of plasma cortisol by dexamethasone.
   d. Loss of stress responsiveness (insulin hypoglycaemia) of plasma cortisol.

N.B. Measurement of plasma ACTH is of no value in the *diagnosis* of Cushing's syndrome, only in the *differential diagnosis*.

apparent on plain abdominal x-ray or intravenous urography. Malignant tumours tend to be bigger (> 100 g) and also tend to secrete a greater proportion of androgens: women are more virilised and 17-OS levels are high. In any cortisol-secreting adrenal tumour, plasma ACTH is suppressed and for this reason the patient has no ACTH-type pigmentation. Rarely, primary adrenal disease is manifested by bilateral nodular hyperplasia of the cortices.

b. Pituitary-dependent Cushing's disease

This is the commonest cause of spontaneous Cushing's syndrome in adults. It is not clear how often the primary fault is a small autonomous adenoma in the pituitary, and how often the increased secretion of pituitary ACTH is secondary to a hypothalamic defect. However, increasing experience with trans-sphenoidal surgery suggests that more than 75% of patients have a pituitary adenoma. Differentiation from the ectopic ACTH syndrome can be very difficult because the pituitary fossa is rarely enlarged on skull x-ray. Plasma ACTH at 08.00h is usually normal or only slightly elevated.

c. Ectopic ACTH syndrome

The majority of cases occur in patients with small cell (oat-cell) lung cancer (Table 4.8), and the plasma ACTH level is usually markedly elevated. The diagnosis may be suggested by the presence of an obvious primary tumour. Otherwise the best clue is the serum potassium: marked hypokalaemia is rare in pituitary Cushing's disease, but it is the rule in the ectopic ACTH syndrome.

d. Alcohol-induced pseudo-Cushing's syndrome

Some alcoholics have the clinical features of Cushing's syndrome, and may also be found to have suggestive biochemical findings; it has therefore been suggested that overindulgence in alcohol may sometimes cause Cushing's syndrome. The suggestion remains unproven.

Table 4.8

More Common Sources of Ectopic ACTH Secretion

1. Lung. Small cell anaplastic (oat-cell) tumours of the bronchus. Bronchial carcinoid tumours.
2. Carcinoid tumours in other foregut derivatives: thymus, pancreas.
3. Tumours of neuroectodermal origin: medullary carcinoma of the thyroid, phaeochromocytoma.
4. Other situations (rare), e.g. ovary.

e. Iatrogenic Cushing's syndrome

As ACTH is now rarely used in therapy, the usual cause is from systemic corticosteroid treatment. Sometimes, however, sufficient steroid may be absorbed from skin application to cause the condition. The diagnosis should be obvious from the history. In addition, patients with this condition are not hirsute (unless the condition is caused by ACTH therapy) since adrenal androgens are suppressed.

Treatment

Treatment is obviously directed at the cause wherever possible. Successful removal of an adrenal tumour will result in complete cure but this is rarely, if ever, achieved in patients with carcinoma of the adrenal. Blood-borne metastases occur and, even if they are not apparent at the time of adrenalectomy, will usually result in the patient's death within two years. Such metastases may be controlled for a time, however, by local irradiation and by treatment with the adrenolytic drug, mitotane (o,pDDD).

There are several approaches to the treatment of pituitary-dependent Cushing's disease but none is consistently successful: they include trans-sphenoidal pituitary surgery, and irradiation either by linear accelerator or by implantation of radioactive Yttrium needles. Some have advocated lowering ACTH secretion by use of centrally-acting drugs such as cyproheptadine or bromocriptine, but most have found that these drugs are only rarely of value.

Attempts to lower ACTH secretion may be unsuccessful, or their full effects may be delayed, and it may therefore be necessary to reduce adrenal steroid secretion directly. This can be done by performing a bilateral adrenalectomy and giving replacement therapy, or by the use of metyrapone or aminoglutethimide – drugs which block cortisol synthesis (Fig. 4.11). There is no place for partial (subtotal) adrenalectomy.

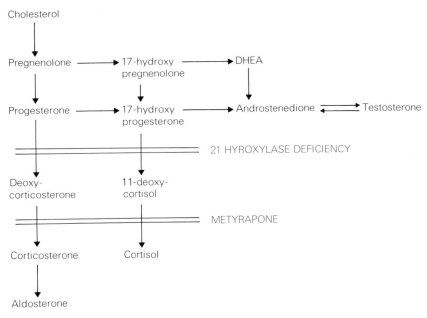

Fig. 4.11 *The effect of metyrapone is to block 11-β-hydroxylase and hence the secretion of cortisol. The negative feedback control increases ACTH secretion and this stimulates an increased secretion of all steroids prior to the enzyme block. 21-hydroxylase deficiency is the commonest cause of congenital adrenal hyperplasia.*

Nelson's syndrome

Some 20–30% of patients with pituitary-dependent Cushing's disease will develop Nelson's syndrome following bilateral adrenalectomy. The removal of the source of the glucocorticoids releases the pituitary from restraint by negative feedback, and the adenoma starts to enlarge. In these cases the pituitary tumour may expand rapidly and the very high levels of ACTH will produce deep pigmentation of the skin. The incidence is reduced by giving irradiation to the pituitary at, or soon after, the time of adrenalectomy.

Conn's Syndrome

Aetiology

If hyperaldosteronism is associated with suppressed levels of renin, it is termed 'primary' or 'idiopathic' and the patient is said to have Conn's syndrome. Histological examination of the adrenal glands may show an adenoma of the zona glomerulosa, or hyperplasia, or both. Carcinoma is exceedingly rare.

Clinical signs and symptoms

Conn's syndrome is thought to account for between 0.1 and 1.0% of all cases of hypertension, and the diagnosis should be seriously considered in any patient with high blood pressure who is found to have hypokalaemia. The differential diagnosis includes those who have hypokalaemia because of diuretic therapy, Cushing's syndrome and other causes unrelated to hypertension. Eating large quantities of liquorice may also simulate this syndrome.

In addition to hypertension, the patient may have symptoms of hypokalaemia such as muscle weakness or polyuria. If there is an adenoma present it is normally small (< 2 cm diameter) and will not be palpable.

Diagnosis

The diagnosis of primary hyperaldosteronism in a patient with hypertension and hypokalaemia is made by demonstrating elevation of plasma aldosterone in association with consistently suppressed levels of renin. Sampling for these substances requires special care and should be undertaken only in consultation with the Department of Chemical Pathology. Samples need to be taken under controlled conditions of posture, and the patient should not have received interfering drugs (e.g. spironolactone, β-blockers) for at least 4 weeks beforehand.

Localisation

Larger adenomas may be seen on CT scan of the abdomen. Sometimes localisation requires selective catheterisation of the adrenal veins with sampling for aldosterone. Adenomas can also be demonstrated by an adrenal isotope scan using radiolabelled cholesterol.

Treatment

If only one gland is involved, unilateral adrenalectomy will reverse the hyperaldosteronism and the hypertension may be cured. Bilateral adrenalectomy, however, is not indicated in patients who have hyperplasia. In such patients the hyperaldosteronism and hypertension can usually be controlled with large doses (up to 400 mg daily) of an aldosterone antagonist such as spironolactone. The same drug can be used as preparation for surgery in any patient with a Conn's adenoma in whom the hypertension and hypokalaemic alkalosis are not otherwise easily treated.

Congenital Adrenal Hyperplasia

Aetiology

This autosomal recessive condition is characterised by deficiency of one of the enzymes necessary for the synthesis of cortisol. The commonest defect is that of 21-hydroxylase (see Fig. 4.11).

Clinical

If the defect is marked, the untreated child with 21-hydroxylase deficiency will die soon after birth from salt and water depletion. However, many forms are partial and if the condition is unrecognised, affected children may survive to adulthood. The effect of the enzyme block is deficient production of cortisol (and, often, aldosterone: *salt-losing* type). Pituitary ACTH secretion rises to overcome the block, and this induces adrenal hyperplasia, and excessive production of precursors including androgens.

If there is sufficient glucocorticoid and mineralocorticoid circulating to enable the undiagnosed child to survive, the dominant clinical effect will be caused by the excessive androgens: girls are virilised at birth with an enlarged clitoris; they grow rapidly to be taller and stronger than any of their friends in the early years of life. However, their epiphyses fuse early and their final height is short (less than five feet). Breasts develop but menstruation is absent or infrequent and adult women remain grossly virilised. Boys undergo a similar early rapid development of height and strength with enlargement of the penis and with pubic and axillary hair growth, but their testes remain small (precocious pseudopuberty). Their final adult height is also stunted but they may be otherwise normal.

The clinical picture in the other enzyme deficiencies differs from that of the 21-hydroxylase and depends on the pattern of corticosteroids produced.

Treatment

As congenital adrenal hyperplasia is a condition of adrenocortical hypofunction, treatment is with glucocorticoid (hydrocortisone, dexamethasone or prednisolone) replacement. It may, in addition, be necessary to give fludrocortisone depending on the degree of aldosterone deficiency. The dose of steroid given has to be adjusted to the individual's size and needs, and this can be difficult to determine: too little renders the child hypoadrenal but too much will produce a Cushingoid state and will stunt final adult height. It is relatively easy to ensure that *enough* is being given by determining full suppression of plasma ACTH, 17-OH-progesterone or urinary pregnanetriol (metabolite of 17-OH-progesterone), but the only reliable way to ensure against overtreatment is by carefully monitoring the child's growth rate.

Boys who receive treatment from birth will develop normally, but girls may require some corrective surgery for clitoromegaly.

5

The Gonads

INTRODUCTION

The primary function of the gonads (ovaries and testes) is to produce their gametes (ova and spermatozoa respectively) and to regulate function of the reproductive tract and sexual behaviour so as to maximise the chances of successful reproduction of the species. With the development of increasingly specialised forms of sexual reproduction in higher vertebrates came the need to evolve a specialised chromosome pair for the control of gonadal differentiation and so of sex differentiation. In mammals these chromosomes are termed X and Y. The heterogametic sex, that is the sex with two different sex chromosomes in each cell, is the male, and the homogametic sex the female. In birds, in contrast, the female is the heterogametic sex. The Y chromo-

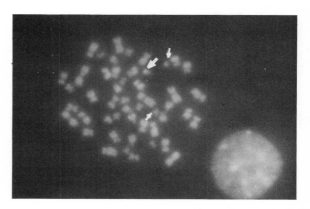

Fig. 5.2 *Quinacrine fluorescence metaphase (left) and interphase (right) nuclei. The cell and nuclear membranes have been disrupted in the former but not in the latter. Small arrows show G-group chromosomes (21 and 22), large arrow shows the Y chromosome with the distal portion of the long arm fluorescing. Large dot in the interphase nucleus is probably the fluorescent Y chromosome.*

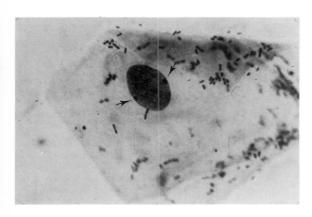

Fig. 5.1 *Buccal smear from a male baby with XXXY karyotype. Arrows show two X chromatin bodies (Barr bodies) in nucleus of the cell. (The squame is covered with lactobacilli.)*

some which controls gonadal differentiation in mammals has become very small, and appears to have lost most of its other non-sex controlling genes. In contrast, much of the genetic material on the X chromosome codes for processes required by both sexes. In order to compensate for what would be an intolerable two-fold difference in X chromosome gene dosage between the sexes, a mechanism has evolved for the random inactivation in all but the gonadal germ cells, of one or other X chromosome. In normal males, in contrast, it is the Y chromosome that is inactivated in somatic cells. The inactivated X chromosome forms the so-called Barr body adjacent to the nuclear membrane in female cells; when the cell undergoes mitotic division this X chromosome divides later than the other chromosomes. Where more than the normal complement of X chromosomes is present, there will be one fewer Barr bodies than there are X chromosomes (Fig. 5.1).

The sex chromosome make-up of an individual, normally XX or XY, is termed the genotypic sex. This in turn determines the apparent physical sex of the individual, termed the phenotypic or body sex. The basic phenotypic sex is female; all that is required for its development is the absence of a Y chromosome. On the other hand, the presence of a Y chromosome early *in utero* leads to the expression of an antigen called the HY antigen (Fig. 5.2). The production of this glycoprotein component of cell walls in male individuals is

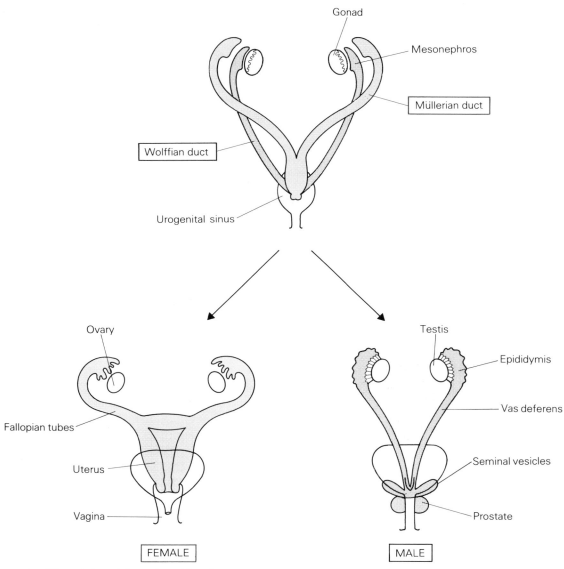

Fig. 5.3 *The differentiation of the male and female.*

dictated by the Y chromosome but apparently also requires the active participation of the X chromosome.

Early in development the primordial germ cells migrate from the endoderm of the yolk sac to the primitive gonad in the urogenital ridge. The arrival of germ cells is essential for further gonadal development. In male fetuses, production of the HY antigen is associated with development of epithelial cords, which later become seminiferous tubules and, at about 8 weeks, the interstitial cells of Leydig. The testes and ovaries are recognisably different by about 6 weeks' gestation.

PRIMARY SEX DIFFERENTIATION

The mechanism in outline appears to be extremely simple (Fig. 5.3). The underlying phenotype is female, and maleness has to be imposed upon it. By about the 8th week of intra-uterine life two pairs of potential reproductive tracts have developed that link the gonads to the urogenital sinus. These are the Müllerian and Wolffian ducts. From around the ninth week the testes produce a polypeptide which causes regression of the Müllerian ducts. In the absence of testes, the

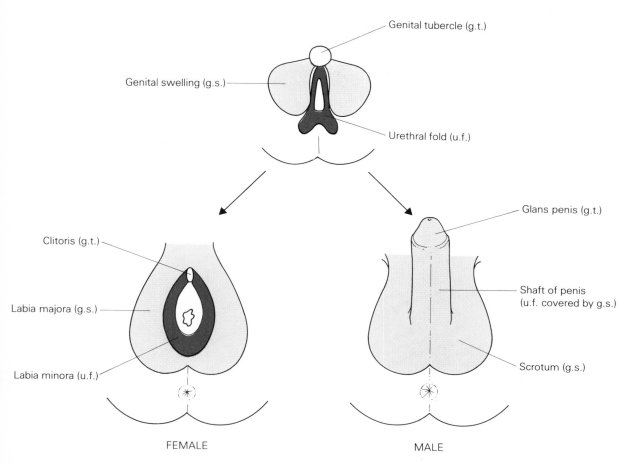

Fig. 5.4 *The development of male and female external genitalia.*

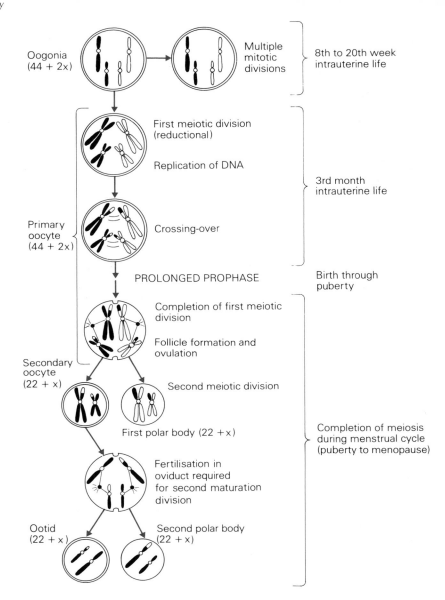

Oogonia
(44 + 2x)

Multiple
mitotic
divisions

8th to 20th week
intrauterine life

First meiotic division
(reductional)

Replication of DNA

3rd month
intrauterine life

Primary
oocyte
(44 + 2x)

Crossing-over

PROLONGED PROPHASE

Birth through
puberty

Completion of first meiotic
division

Follicle formation and
ovulation

Secondary
oocyte
(22 + x)

Second meiotic division

First polar body (22 + x)

Completion of meiosis
during menstrual cycle
(puberty to menopause)

Fertilisation in
oviduct required
for second maturation
division

Ootid
(22 + x)

Second polar body
(22 + x)

Fig. 5.5 (a) The meiotic process in germ cells in the female at different stages of sexual development.

Müllerian ducts persist and develop to form the female internal genitalia (uterus and Fallopian tubes). A little later, there is increasing production of testosterone by the Leydig cells, which are stimulated by the placental hormone human chorionic gonadotrophin (HCG). The

Wolffian ducts are hormone-dependent and require exposure to testosterone in order to persist. The external, in contrast to the internal, genitalia are developed from the same structures in both sexes, namely the genital tubercle, urethral folds and genital

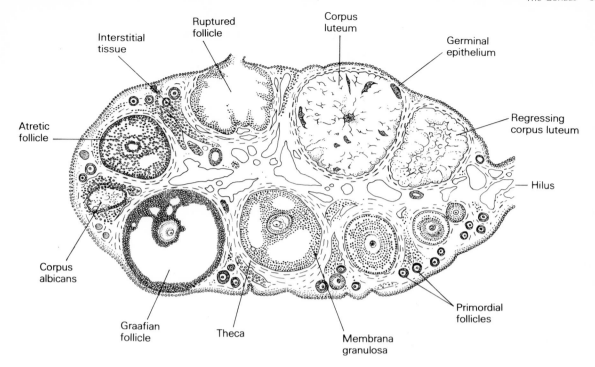

Fig. 5.5 *(b) Follicle and corpus luteum development within the ovary.*

swellings (Fig. 5.4). The major factor promoting male differentiation of the external genitalia is androgen produced by the testis; testosterone secreted by the testis is first converted by a tissue enzyme 5α-reductase, to dihydrotestosterone (DHT) which is the active androgen in these structures. Around term the testes, again by a mechanism involving the action of testosterone on the gubernacula, descend with their associated structures to their final place in the scrotal sac.

Androgens act on tissues in a way that is similar to that of other steroid hormones. To be effective the organ must make specific protein molecules ('receptors') which bind to the steroid, move into the nucleus and there bind to specific regions of DNA. This apparently allows selected specific genes to be 'read' by the enzyme RNA polymerase. Messenger RNA produced is translated into protein synthesis (including more receptor) in the cytoplasm.

In the ovary between the 8th and 20th week of intrauterine life, primitive oogonia divide repeatedly, and then start to undergo meiotic division to form the oocytes (Fig. 5.5a). These are surrounded by granulosa cells to become primordial follicles (Fig. 5.5b). The oocytes are apparently held in this suppressed state by their surrounding follicular cells. At this stage the ovary appears to have no control over events in other related tissues.

Abnormalities in Primary Sex Differentiation

There are numerous places where the above processes can go wrong, and many abnormalities have been described. It is important for the student to understand the basic principles outlined above, which are well illustrated if we consider some of these disorders.

Gonadal dysgenesis

In its pure form the gonad fails to develop altogether. The individual has degenerate 'streak' gonads, and whether the genetic sex is XY or XX, the internal and external genital tract structures are female. The patient will usually present complaining of failure of menstruation (primary amenorrhoea) at the time of normal puberty. There is nothing that can be done to make such women fertile, but they will have withdrawal bleeding in response to cyclical hormone therapy. In the future such women wishing pregnancy will doubtless be suitable hosts for donor fertilised ova. The condition is rare. Less rare is Turner's syndrome, which is usually caused by the loss of an X or Y chromosome in the fertilised ovum. These individuals have a similar complaint of amenorrhoea, but are usually short and show other abnormalities such as webbing of the neck, increased carrying angle, widely spaced nipples and cardiovascular abnormalities such as coarctation of the aorta (Fig. 5.6).

Testicular feminisation

This is a rare X-linked disorder due to a defective gene coding for the androgen receptor. No matter how much androgen the tissues are exposed to, normal

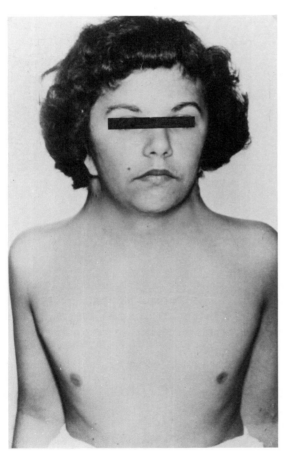

Fig. 5.6 *Clinical features of Turner's syndrome (XO gonadal dysgenesis). Note webbing of the neck and widely-spaced nipples.*

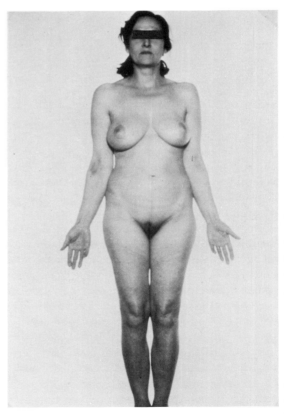

Fig. 5.7 *Testicular feminisation. Note normal female breast development and lack of secondary sexual hair. Patient had testes palpable in the labia.*

androgen target organs are unable to respond. Therefore, in an affected male fetus *in utero* the Wolffian ducts disappear, and the external genitalia develop along female lines. On the other hand, Müllerian duct inhibition occurs as expected, and so the individual does not develop a uterus or Fallopian tubes. The testes remain either in the inguinal canals or the labia. At the time of normal puberty such individuals develop breasts because the testes produce oestrogens as well as androgens. In the classical form they do not develop sexual (pubic or axillary) hair, which is also androgen-dependent (Fig. 5.7). Such patients must obviously be raised as females, and later in life (after puberty), the testes should be removed because of a risk of tumour development. Females carry the condition, but do not express it, presumably because of the normal gene present on the second X chromosome and the relatively trivial effects of androgens in the female.

5α-reductase deficiency

In this rare autosomal recessive disorder there is a failure to convert testosterone to dihydrotestosterone which, as discussed already, is the important androgen in some target tissues. The internal genitalia are those of a normal male, but the external genitalia do not virilise properly. Affected boys are raised as females, but show signs of virilisation with growth of the phallus and male sexual behaviour at the time of puberty. The voice deepens, but there is usually scanty facial and body hair.

True hermaphroditism

It is difficult to generalise about the abnormalities which result, for example, if one gonad is a testis and the other an ovary, as a result of one gonad containing a Y chromosome and the other not. These conditions are very rare and highly varied.

Primary virilisation in a genetic female (see also Chapter 3)

The commonest cause is an enzyme defect in the adrenal glands, most often 21-hydroxylase deficiency. This condition is inherited as an autosomal recessive and occurs once in about 7000 births. The 21-hydroxylase defect impairs the production of cortisol and

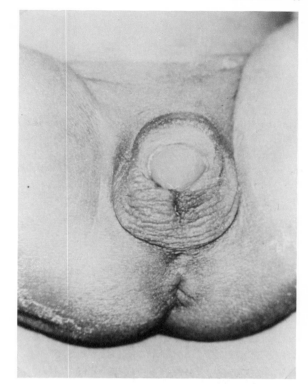

Fig. 5.8 *External virilisation with clitoromegaly and labioscrotal fusion in a female infant with congenital adrenal hyperplasia secondary to 21-hydroxylase deficiency.*

hence ACTH levels rise. Excessive amounts of 17α-hydroxyprogesterone, and the androgenic by-products androstenedione and testosterone, are produced. In female infants in whom excessive androgen production has occurred from an early stage *in utero*, there may be an extreme degree of external virilisation, with the external genitalia resembling those of the normal male, but usually with the urethra opening at the base of the penis (hypospadias) (Fig. 5.8). In milder cases the scrotum is not fused, and there is simply some clitoral enlargement. Aldosterone in addition is not produced in adequate amounts in about a third of cases, in which event the infant rapidly develops severe salt loss and dehydration. This is most likely to be fatal in boys in whom there is no apparent genital abnormality to alert the doctor. Treatment is with replacement adrenal steroids.

Intersexual states later in life

There are many minor intersexual disorders, such as isolated hypospadias in males, whose causes are unknown. Sometimes minor enzyme defects are not recognised at birth and are only present at the time of normal puberty. Their precise diagnosis is for the specialist, and depends on detailed biochemical analysis.

SEXUAL MATURATION

After birth there is a prolonged period of relative gonadal inactivity, which ends with the onset of

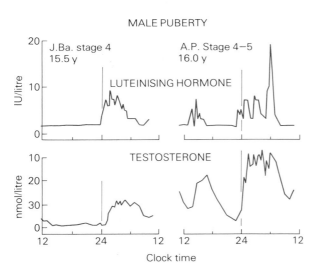

Fig. 5.9 *Luteinising hormone (LH) and testosterone levels in two boys with delayed, but otherwise normal, puberty. Note episodic secretion of both hormones, initially starting at night time but later extending to the daytime period. The rise in testosterone is secondary to that of LH. (After Large and Anderson, 1979.)*

puberty. These changes are apparently triggered by central brain mechanisms which result in the episodic stimulation of the cells of the pituitary gland by gonadotrophin releasing hormone (GnRH) from the hypothalamus. This substance is a decapeptide which has now been isolated and synthesised (see Chapter 2). The first hormone changes are a rise in night-time levels of luteinising hormone (LH) and, to a lesser extent, follicle stimulating hormone (FSH), which are produced in episodic bursts (Fig. 5.9). These hormones act through receptors which activate adenylate cyclase on specific cells in the gonads.

Male Puberty

As LH rises progressively, first during sleep, and later in the daytime as well, the Leydig cells produce increasing amounts of testosterone. Plasma levels of this hormone rise more than twenty-fold during puberty. At the same time the cells of the seminiferous tubules (germ cells and supporting Sertoli cells) mature, and the complicated process of spermatogenesis progresses with the continuous production of large numbers of spermatozoa (Fig. 5.10). The testes enlarge, mainly due to growth of the seminiferous tubules (Fig. 5.11). Stimulated by LH, the Leydig cells secrete testosterone which acts locally on the tubules and, in combination with FSH, stimulates spermatogenesis (Fig. 5.12). Testosterone is also secreted into the spermatic veins, and travels in the blood stream throughout the body where it acts on susceptible tissues. It is responsible directly, or after conversion to dihydrotestosterone, for secondary sexual changes such as enlargement of the larynx and deepening of the voice, enlargement of penis, scrotum, prostate, seminal vesicles, epididymis and vas deferens, and stimulation of sexual behaviour. Secondary sexual hair is also androgen-dependent, although it evidently varies a great deal in extent between different individuals, and between different races. Parts of the autonomic nervous system concerned with erection and ejaculation appear to be androgen-dependent.

The testes in turn exert some controlling negative feedback effect on the hypothalamus and pituitary, although this is much less dramatic than in the case of the ovaries (see below). Spermatogenesis may be associated with a factor (inhibin) that selectively reduces the production by pituitary cells of FSH.

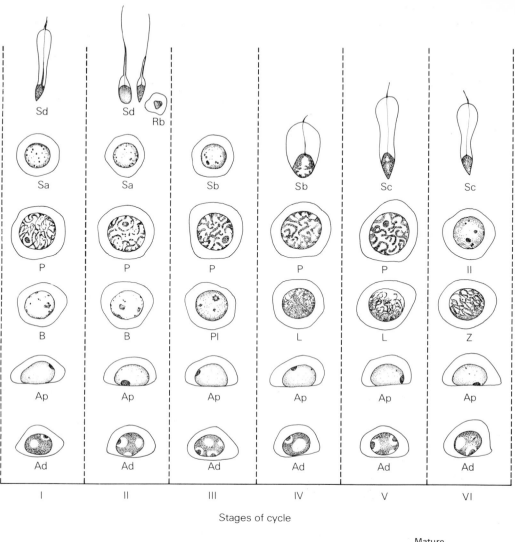

Stages of cycle

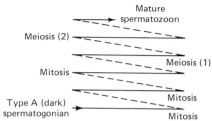

Fig. 5.10 *Comparison of six cellular associations (I–VI) observed in seminiferous epithelium of man. Transformation into spermatozoa from type A spermatogonia can be followed by reading along from left to right, starting at bottom row. Ad = dark type A spermatogonia; Ap = pale type A spermatogonia; B = type B spermatogonia: primary spermatocytes;*

PL = preleptotene; L = leptotene; Z = zygotene; P = pachytene; II = secondary spermatocyte; Sa − Sd = steps in final maturation of spermatozoa; Rb = residual body. 'Dark' and 'pale' refer to appearance on staining. (After Clermont Y. (1966) Fertil. Steril., 17, 705.)

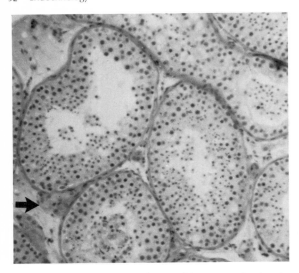

Fig. 5.11 *Gross appearance of normal human testis, showing tubules (cut across) and Leydig cells (arrowed).*

Female Puberty and the Onset of Ovulation and Menstruation

Similar central mechanisms initiate gonadotrophin secretion in girls. Stimulation of the ovary by FSH is necessary for follicles to mature and release the ovum. We do not know the precise mechanisms which select a particular single follicle for 'ripening'. Initially a group of follicles mature together, and produce oestrogen. Early in puberty many cycles may occur without ovulation. Finally one follicle 'takes off' and enlarges progressively to a diameter of more than two centimetres. This enlargement is caused by a massive increase in the number of cells in the follicle — cells of the theca interna, and granulosa cells (Fig. 5.5b) — and the secretion of fluid into the antrum of the follicle.

Androgens produced in the theca interna are converted to the oestrogens, oestrone and oestradiol, by the granulosa cells lining the follicle wall. While this process is occurring, the ovum itself is undergoing the later stages of meiotic division, in preparation for fertilisation if coitus occurs. A marked rise in blood oestrogen level occurs during the five days prior to ovulation (Fig. 5.13). This rise in oestrogen exerts a marked effect on the pituitary, making it more sensitive to GnRH, and probably on the hypothalamus, simultaneously suppressing GnRH production. When the follicle is fully mature, the oestrogen production falls and progesterone starts to rise; these two changes trigger the hypothalamus to discharge prolonged and massive bursts of GnRH, leading to massive episodic rises in LH level in the blood. It is this LH surge which, acting on the follicle, finally causes it to rupture (Fig. 5.14) with release of the ovum and transformation of the granulosa cells into the corpus luteum (Fig. 5.5b).

The second half of the menstrual cycle is dominated, from an endocrine point of view, by the corpus luteum, whose principal role is to secrete large amounts of progesterone. Together with secreted oestradiol, this acts on a variety of tissues, the most important of which is the uterus. Oestradiol secreted by the follicle has prepared the endometrium by producing glandular growth — the so-called proliferative phase. An important effect of oestrogens is to induce the production of cytoplasmic receptors for progesterone; these allow the endometrium to respond in a way outlined above for androgens, to the high progesterone levels produced by the corpus luteum. The structure of the endometrium is converted from proliferative to secretory, in preparation for implantation of an embryo. In that event, the hormone human chorionic gonadotrophin (HCG) produced by the implanted trophoblast stimulates and sustains the corpus luteum, which in turn produces sufficient progesterone to maintain the endometrium during early pregnancy.

Menstruation occurs if pregnancy has not resulted, when the corpus luteum succumbs to its natural lifespan, and progesterone levels fall. As progesterone levels fall, secretion by endometrial cells diminishes, the endometrium collapses, and the spiral arteries shrink. The surface layers of endometrium die from lack of blood supply and are shed. Meanwhile a new crop of follicles starts to enlarge and produce oestrogen, and one is 'selected' for ovulation; the next menstrual cycle begins.

The most obvious secondary sexual change accompanying female puberty is the development of breasts; many hormones act upon the breast, the most important being oestradiol, which stimulates epithelial proliferation. The epithelium in turn probably stimulates local fat-cell growth which is responsible for most of the

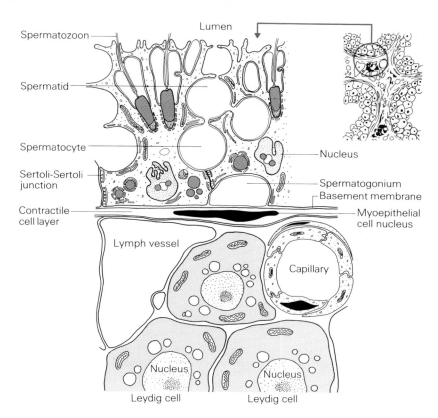

Fig. 5.12 *Diagram of normal testis to show relationship between Sertoli cells, germ cells (inside tubules) and Leydig cells (outside tubules). Spermatogonia and spermatocytes occupy the spaces indicated.*

increase in breast size. Progesterone also acts, though only on the 'oestrogen-primed' breast, causing an increase in breast volume. Prolactin from the pituitary is important only in stimulating milk secretion necessary for the suckling infant. Levels rise under the stimulus of high levels of oestrogen during pregnancy where oestrogens also block its effect on the breast and by neural reflex mechanisms during suckling. Oestrogens also stimulate long bone growth, and closure of the epiphyses, so that growth is ultimately arrested.

Many of the secondary characteristics that differentiate the sexes result from the effect of high levels of androgens in men and their absence in women. An example is the breast; there is ample oestrogen secreted by the normal male to stimulate breast development if this process were not antagonised in some way that is not fully understood by testosterone. A particularly obvious example of this is the marked breast development that occurs, under the influence of testicular oestrogen, when tissues have an inborn resistance to androgens (testicular feminisation). Small amounts of androgen are produced in women from the ovaries (where they are essential for oestrogen synthesis), and in both sexes from the adrenals — these lead to the development of secondary sexual hair, the adrenarche.

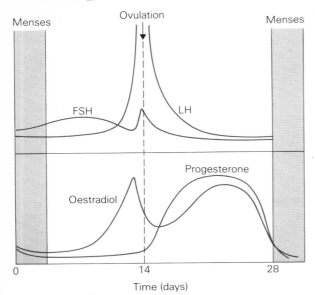

Fig. 5.13 *Pattern of hormone release during the normal menstrual cycle.*

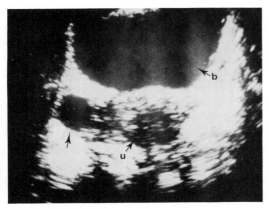

Fig. 5.14 *Ultrasound scan of pelvis at the time of ovulation. Plain arrow indicates a normal follicle (right ovary) 2 cm in diameter just before ovulation. b = bladder; u = uterus.*

DISORDERS OF SECONDARY SEX DIFFERENTIATION

Gynaecomastia in Men

Men possess vestigial breast tissue which is capable of responding to the right hormonal milieu; this consists of either an increase in oestrogen level, a decrease in androgen level or both. Transient gynaecomastia is a normal accompaniment of male puberty, where the oestradiol level rises proportionately more than testosterone in the early stages. This oestradiol is in part secreted by the testis, and in part produced in peripheral tissues from testosterone. In androgen deficiency from any cause (see below) gynaecomastia is common. Some drugs, such as digoxin, spironolactone, cyproterone acetate and cimetidine have oestrogenic and/or anti-androgenic effects which disturb the process of breast inhibition in men. Feminising tumours of testis or adrenal are other rare causes. Oestrogens are still administered for treatment of carcinoma of prostate, with inevitable gynaecomastia. Gynaecomastia occurs in some patients with cirrhosis, and also with thyrotoxicosis. In both conditions there is increased SHBG production, which plays a role in the change of oestrogen-androgen balance. Rarely, bronchial carcinomas may secrete human chorionic gonadotrophin which stimulates interstitial cells to produce androgens and oestrogens. Gynaecomastia is also found in patients with hypogonadism (e.g. Klinefelter's syndrome, post castration, hypopituitarism).

Gynaecomastia is common in old age, probably due to reduced production of testosterone whilst oestradiol production remains relatively unchanged.

The treatment of gynaecomastia depends first of all on identifying its cause. Mild pubertal gynaecomastia requires no treatment. Drugs without feminising effects can be substituted if this is the cause. For hypogonadism, androgens are often an effective treatment. However, even if a cause can be found and effectively treated, the breast changes may not resolve and mastectomy via a periareolar incision is required.

Hirsutism in Women

The borderline between physiological increase in secondary sexual hair in women and pathological hirsutism is an arbitrary one. Most women with a definite increase in facial hair have an increased production of testosterone. Testosterone circulates predominantly bound to plasma proteins, of which the principal one is sex-hormone-binding globulin (SHBG). However it is the unbound fraction which is free to act on the tissues. In most hirsute women SHBG levels are reduced, and although the total testosterone level may be normal its free concentration is increased. The source of testosterone may be the adrenals, the ovaries or both. Some hirsute women have irregular and infrequent menstrual periods although gonadotrophin levels are not reduced; in fact the LH level is often elevated. The ovaries contain multiple cysts, and produce more androgen (testosterone and androstenedione) and less oestrogen than normal (Fig. 5.15). The cause of this polycystic ovary syndrome, which does not always lead to hirsutism, is uncertain. It is commonly associated with infertility, because ovulation is infrequent and erratic. Ovulation can often be induced with the use of antioestrogenic drugs such as clomiphene. These cause a rise in LH and FSH, which stimulate follicle development; the oestrogen produced by a committed follicle may then be sufficient to induce a surge of LH, which causes ovulation as described above.

In addition to 'idiopathic' hirsutism and polycystic ovarian disease there are other causes which, although rare, are important to recognise. They include Cushing's syndrome (see Chapter 4), and late-onset congenital adrenal hyperplasia. The latter can readily be excluded by measuring plasma levels of 17α-hydroxy-progesterone, which are very high. Virilising tumours of ovary or adrenal glands are uncommon and usually benign; they are suspected in cases of rapid onset of severe hirsutism with balding and clitoral enlargement, associated with marked elevation of plasma testosterone (>5 nmol/l, normal <2 nmol/l), androstenedione, and/or dehydroepiandrosterone sulphate (the latter only in adrenal tumours). Modern scanning methods (computer tomography and ultrasound) are very helpful in localising such tumours which, however, account for only a very small percentage of cases of hirsutism. The treatment is surgical removal.

Hirsutism itself may be treated by various combinations of adrenal and ovarian suppression, antiandrogens (for severe cases) and cosmetic therapy — of which the only permanent one is electrolysis.

Adrenal suppression with low-dose prednisolone is indicated in congenital adrenal hyperplasia. In polycystic ovarian disease it sometimes leads to regular ovulation and so may be worth a short therapeutic trial is some cases. For ovarian suppression some oral contraceptives containing androgenic progestogens such as norethisterone or norgestrel are unsuitable for obvious reasons. The best regimes for use in hirsute women combine ethinyl oestradiol with a non-androgenic potent progestogen such as medroxyprogesterone acetate or desogestrel. Cyproterone acetate the potent anti-androgenic progestogen has the disadvantage of a long half-life, which means that it must be given from day 1–10 (100 mg/day), with ethinyl oestradiol (30 µg/day) from day 1–21. If given for longer at high dose there is no withdrawal bleeding when the oestrogen is stopped. Spironolactone has some anti-androgenic (as well as antimineralocorticoid) effect, and is also useful in a dose of 100–200 mg/day, for example after the menopause or where oestrogens are contra-indicated.

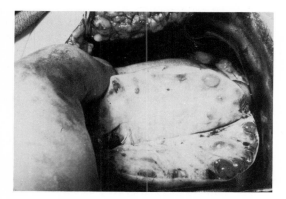

Fig. 5.15 *Gross surgical appearance of a large polycystic ovary.*

Hypogonadism in Men

As part of the process of ageing there is some decline both in hormone production from the testis and in spermatogenesis. This does not usually occur in men until after the age of 50, and is highly variable in onset and degree. Since oestrogen production is well maintained, mild gynaecomastia may develop as a normal accompaniment of ageing. The term 'hypogonadism' in the male is generally used to imply defective androgen production, and consequent clinical signs of androgen deficiency; an almost inevitable accompaniment is impaired sperm production. Conditions causing defective spermatogenesis alone are considered separately below.

Clinical features

Features of androgen deficiency arising *in utero* have already been discussed. Androgen deficiency is of course physiological in childhood. In individuals in whom testosterone is not produced at the time of normal puberty, the long bones continue to grow, albeit slowly, so that the legs are long and final height is increased. Span exceeds height and pubis–heel distance exceeds that of crown-pubis. In addition, normal androgen-induced muscular development is absent, body fat is distributed over bony prominences of the trunk and buttocks, gynaecomastia may be present, the voice does not break and secondary sexual hair is scanty and confined to the pubic triangle and axilla. The penis remains infantile, the scrotum is small and non-pigmented and the prostate impalpable on rectal examination. Erections, nocturnal emissions, masturbation and sexual interest are absent. The testes are small. When androgen deficiency develops after normal puberty, the features are the same except that body proportions are normal, the voice broken and the penis normal in size. The testes will usually be soft.

Causes of hypogonadism

The causes may be conveniently classified according to whether gonadotrophin levels are elevated (hypergonadotrophic) or reduced (hypogonadotrophic). The former consists of conditions in which the testis is primarily at fault, the latter where androgen deficiency is secondary to gonadotrophin lack.

Hypergonadotrophic hypogonadism

Klinefelter's syndrome: This is the commonest cause of hypergonadotrophic hypogonadism and is nearly always due to an XXY chromosome constitution. Although primary sex differentiation is normal the germ cells degenerate shortly after birth to leave 'ghost' tubules lined only by Sertoli cells (Fig. 5.16). The testes are therefore very small. Partial puberty usually occurs, and androgen deficiency is seldom complete. The Leydig cells are apparently hypertrophic, occurring in clumps between the ghost tubules; however, despite high levels of LH, they do not produce normal amounts of testosterone. These individuals may present with pubertal failure, gynaecomastia or infertility with azoospermia (Fig. 5.17). A minority are of low intelligence, and behavioural abnormalities are probably no commoner than in other individuals with testicular hormone deficiency. Where androgen deficiency is marked, androgen replacement therapy is indicated (see below).

Late testicular degeneration (anorchia): In these conditions the testes degenerate, for some reason, after the stage of primary sex differentiation. Many other conditions such as drugs, irradiation and viruses such as mumps may damage the testes; generally the germ cells are more susceptible than the Leydig or Sertoli cells. Leydig cells, however, do not function normally when the tubules are severely damaged.

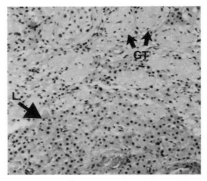

Fig. 5.16 *Testicular biopsy from a patient with Klinefelter's syndrome showing clumps of Leydig cells (L) and ghost tubules (GT) devoid of germ cells.*

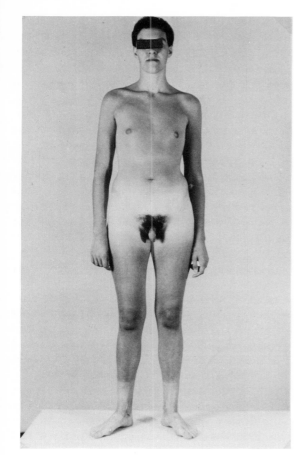

Fig. 5.17 *21-year-old patient with XXY Klinefelter's syndrome. Note long limbs, scanty pubic hair of female distribution, mild gynaecomastia, small testes and underdeveloped scrotum.*

Hypogonadotrophic hypogonadism

Isolated gonadotrophin deficiency: In these individuals there is a failure of gonadotrophin production at the time of normal puberty, which may be complete or partial. In some patients the low levels of gonadotrophin result from an inability to synthesise gonadotrophin-releasing hormone. When associated with absent sense of smell (anosmia), this is termed Kallmann's syndrome and is associated with defective olfactory pathways. In occasional individuals with partial gonadotrophin deficiency, FSH production is normal and spermatogenesis is preserved, while peripheral signs of androgen deficiency occur. In such 'fertile eunuchs' normal virilisation and sperm production can be produced by treatment with human chorionic gonadotrophin alone.

Simple delayed puberty: This cannot usually be distinguished with certainty from permanent isolated gonadotrophin deficiency except in retrospect. Occasionally it is evident that inadequate weight gain has occurred, or the individual has true anorexia nervosa which has produced regression back to prepubertal gonadotrophin levels.

Hypopituitarism: Often other features, such as hypothyroidism or adrenal insufficiency are apparent. Important clinical pointers are a complaint of headaches, visual field defects due to pressure on the optic chiasm, short stature due to growth hormone deficiency (this only occurs if GH secretion is lost during childhood or adolescence) and absence or reduction of secondary sexual hair (Fig. 5.18). Occasionally, galactorrhoea is complained of or may be revealed on examining the breasts; in such cases, prolactin levels are usually elevated. Hypopituitarism may be caused by a wide variety of lesions, and is discussed in Chapter 2.

Treatment of hypogonadism

Infertility due to gonadotrophin deficiency can be treated with HCG, 1500 units twice weekly, combined with FSH therapy. Pergonal is a combination of LH and FSH; it is extremely expensive and therefore only justified for a trial period in a gonadotrophin-deficient man in whom fertility is urgently desired. An alternative treatment currently being used is the pulsatile administration of gonadotrophin-releasing hormone (GnRH) using a portable minipump. This is only applicable when there are gonadotrophs in the pituitary capable of being stimulated. Sex hormone replacement is discussed on p. 99.

Low sperm count, without hypogonadism

The vast majority of men with infertility do not have any impairment of androgen production by the testes. Many have problems unrelated to spermatogenesis

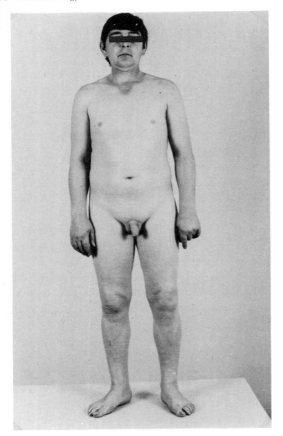

Fig. 5.18 *45-year-old man with panhypopituitarism which had developed over the preceding 5 years due to a very large prolactinoma. Note complete loss of secondary sexual hair, normal body proportions.*

directly, or involving the later stages of maturation, which occur outside the testes in the epididymes. In others, subtle factors such as raised scrotal temperature damage spermatogenesis. However, in some men, unknown factors have produced a variable degree of selective damage to the germ cells, causing the so-called Sertoli-cell-only syndrome. FSH levels are high in such men.

Hypogonadism in Women

Hypergonadotrophic hypogonadism

Physiological–menopause: The normal menopause generally takes place at around the age of 50. The total number of follicles is determined shortly after birth and, even in childhood, progressively more degenerate to produce a fibrosed remnant (an atretic follicle). After puberty a cohort of follicles becomes committed each cycle; one is selected to ovulate, and the rest degenerate. Once the supply is exhausted, levels of oestradiol (and progesterone) fall, and gonadotrophin levels (LH and FSH) rise. There are commonly symptoms of oestrogen deficiency (vaginal dryness, loss of libido) combined with episodic hot flushes, when there is sudden generalised vasodilatation. The mechanisms of the latter are not known but they are relieved, in part at least, with low doses of oestrogens, and often gradually improve without treatment. Hot flushes coincide with peaks of gonadotrophin secretion, but are not caused by them.

Pathological: Pure gonadal dysgenesis and Turner's syndrome have been discussed above. In both, primary amenorrhoea, failure of breast development and high circulating gonadotrophin levels are associated with streak gonads. In pure gonadal dysgenesis the phenotype is otherwise normal, while Turner's syndrome is suggested by short stature, low hairline, widely-spaced nipples, and sometimes a webbed neck, lymphoedema, and cardiovascular abnormalities such as coarctation of the aorta. The chromosome count is usually 45 XO, and can be readily checked by peripheral blood leucocyte culture.

Hypergonadotrophic hypogonadism may develop after pelvic irradiation or chemotherapy for leukaemia in childhood. Premature menopause may arise from production of anti-ovarian antibodies, although usually the cause is unknown, and may simply be a low initial number of follicles. Affected patients present with secondary amenorrhoea.

Hypogonadotrophic hypogonadism

The female is particularly susceptible to disturbances of hypothalamic control of gonadotrophin production associated with psychiatric disorders or loss of weight. Anorexia nervosa is a common condition with pathological dieting, weight loss and a disturbed body image. It is almost invariably accompanied by amenorrhoea and hypogonadism, usually in a girl who has already menstruated (i.e. secondary amenorrhoea). It is necessary for a female to reach a critical body weight before ovulation can commence and weight-loss from any cause may lead to amenorrhoea. Treatment of the hypogonadism is directed at the primary condition in the first instance.

Hyperprolactinaemia is much commoner in women than in men. Oestrogens stimulate production of this hormone, and benign prolactin-secreting pituitary tumours (prolactinomas) arise much more frequently in women. In addition to galactorrhoea these cause amenorrhoea, in part by inhibition of hypothalamic GnRH release and in part by a direct inhibitory effect on the ovary. In fact, basal circulating gonadotrophin levels are often normal unless the pituitary tumour is very large. Normal reproductive function usually results when prolactin levels are lowered with the dopamine agonist bromocriptine. Many drugs which either deplete dopamine stores or antagonise the effects of dopamine stimulate prolactin production, which is normally under inhibitory control from hypothalamic dopamine.

Another cause of hypogonadotrophic hypogonadism in the female is isolated gonadotrophin deficiency; the diagnosis is usually made by a process of exclusion although, as with men, some affected women have anosmia (Kallman's syndrome). Craniopharyngioma is the most likely tumour in the region of the pituitary to cause primary amenorrhoea, because of its relatively high incidence in childhood.

In women in whom it is desired to restore fertility and menstruation, the solution is relatively simple for those with hyperprolactinaemia and normal gonadotrophin reserve. Measures to lower prolactin, usually involving treatment with bromocriptine, are rapidly effective even in women with large pituitary tumours. There is a small but significant risk of tumour enlargement during pregnancy. For this reason, in an infertile woman seeking pregnancy, the treatment should be supervised in a specialised centre, particularly if the pituitary fossa is expanded on x-ray. Usually, bromocriptine is stopped once the woman is pregnant but, should a visual field defect develop it should be restarted immediately. In women with permanent gonadotrophin deficiency it is usually necessary to give injections of LH and FSH, and to monitor urinary or plasma oestrogens and follicle size by ultrasound, and then to induce ovulation of a 'ripe' follicle by injecting HCG. This treatment is also in the province of the specialist, because of the risks of multiple follicle development and massive ovarian enlargement from hyperstimulation.

Tests of Gonadal Function

A thorough history and clinical examination will usually lead to a provisional diagnosis. In men, a normal sperm count (if masturbation is possible) excludes significant hypogonadism. The next step is to decide whether the gonadotrophin levels are high or low, and to measure prolactin. In women, an important pitfall in interpreting high gonadotrophin levels is the fact that LH is normally high at mid-cycle, and may be modestly raised in the polycystic ovary syndrome. In anyone with amenorrhoea the possibility of pregnancy must be borne in mind and excluded — HCG levels will be high, and this will cause an apparently high LH on radioimmunoassay. Pelvic ultrasound is of value both in excluding pregnancy and in assessing ovarian size.

In both sexes, if the gonadotrophin levels are high a blood karyotype should be carried out. In men, plasma testosterone gives a good measure of the degree of androgen deficiency. Stimulation tests of pituitary gonadotrophin release with GnRH may be helpful in confirming gonadotrophin deficiency. In this event, other tests of pituitary function should include TSH, thyroid hormone levels and, in an otherwise well individual, the response of growth hormone and cortisol to controlled insulin-induced hypoglycaemia. Plain x-rays of the pituitary fossa are mandatory in hypogonadotrophic hypogonadism in both sexes. In women with anorexia nervosa who have gained weight but are still amenorrhoeic, a therapeutic trial of the anti-oestrogen climiphene, (preferably with measurement of gonadotrophin response) may be useful for inducing ovulation. Other stimulation tests (e.g. clomiphene, and HCG in the male) are only rarely useful in diagnosis.

Sex Hormone Replacement

In general, hormone deficiencies should be rectified wherever they are significantly affecting the health or wellbeing of an individual. Wherever practicable it is probably better to use the natural rather than a synthetic hormone. In *men*, androgen deficiency is relatively infrequent; testosterone is usually given as an intramuscular injection of long-acting esters, which leads to a relatively slow release of the hormone over the succeeding 2–3 weeks. Implantation of fused pellets of testosterone, every 4–6 months under the skin of the abdominal wall, leads to steady release of the hormone but requires a minor surgical procedure under local anaesthetic. Testosterone itself is inactivated in the liver if swallowed, but the undecanoate ester is also available as an oral preparation. Most androgen-deficient men are keen to have one or other such treatment in the long term; testosterone replacement enhances wellbeing, restores potency and protects bones from osteoporosis. Androgen deficiency is the only established indication for testosterone therapy. Testosterone replacement is contra-indicated in prostatic cancer.

In *women*, sex hormone replacement is more difficult. All women become oestrogen-deficient from the time of the menopause. It is established that oestrogens protect the bones against postmenopausal osteoporosis. They also correct many of the troublesome symptoms such as intermittent hot flushes, vaginal dryness, reduced libido and urinary frequency that often accompany oestrogen deficiency; they should certainly be given to women with premature ovarian failure, at least until the time of the normal menopause. A practical problem results from the need to produce cyclical shedding of the endometrium by giving a progestogen as well since, if oestrogens are given alone, the endometrium builds up, becomes hyperplastic and irregular 'break-through' bleeding occurs.

Many women are reluctant to accept continuing periods after the time of menopause. In those in whom a hysterectomy has been performed, oestrogens alone can be given, without the above problems. It is likely that over the next decade attitudes of women and their doctors towards hormone replacement therapy (HRT) will change as many more appreciate the improved wellbeing that commonly results, often from the relief of symptoms which the patient had resignedly come to accept as part of ageing.

Oestrogen replacement is generally given as oral synthetic or conjugated oestrogens. Ethinyl oestradiol (10–20 μg/day) is the simplest to use. Every 1–2 months, a progestogen such as norethisterone acetate (5 mg/day) is added for 7–14 days, and bleeding will follow its withdrawal. On this dose the risks of vascular complications are small; as an alternative, oestradiol can be given subcutaneously as an implant of a fused pellet of the pure steroid.

Sex Hormones and Behaviour

We generally ignore the fact that many of the overall differences in male and female behaviour are mediated or influenced by sex hormones. This is clearly apparent in the male if testosterone is suddenly withdrawn by castration; lethargy and depression, and loss of libido and potency, follow rapidly. There is, however, little to support the idea that homosexuality (sexual attraction towards one's own sex) or trans-sexuality (identification with and the sexual desire to change to one of the opposite sex) are mediated in any way by the individual's pattern of sex hormone production, which is generally normal.

Hormones and Premenstrual Tension

Many women experience severe physical and/or emotional symptoms that are apparently clearly related to certain stages of the menstrual cycle. In some, these are worst premenstrually (PMT).

In view of the tumultuous changes in levels of oestradiol and progesterone that accompany the normal cycle it is perhaps surprising that cyclical emotional disturbances are not more common. Since the hormone patterns are not generally different between women with 'PMT' and those without, it seems likely that the hormone fluctuations are serving as the 'trigger' in a 'primed' individual. Treatments, for which varying success is claimed, include pyridoxine, the 'pill', and progesterone by suppository or injection.

GONADAL TUMOURS

Testicular Tumours

About 1% of malignant neoplasms in man arise in the

testis, and almost all are of germ-cell origin. These include embryonal cell carcinoma, seminoma, choriocarcinoma and teratomas. Most present with enlargement of the testis, but some are in addition hormonally active, producing HCG. Interstitial cell tumours are rare and usually benign; they may secrete oestrogens and cause feminisation. The early recognition of malignant tumours of the testis is important; with effective treatment the prognosis is relatively good, although if untreated they are highly malignant.

Ovarian Tumours

The classification of ovarian tumours is extremely confused. They may be classified according to gross morphology (e.g. solid or cystic), according to their cell or structure of origin, and according to their clinical effects. There are five main groups: serosal; sex-cord stromal; germ cell; metastatic tumours; and miscellaneous. Those that are endocrinologically active are usually sex-cord stromal. The commonest of these are the granulosa cell tumours, which account for 1–2% of ovarian cancers and 5–10% of all ovarian tumours; they are often bilateral, and secrete oestrogens. The clinical presentation in the child is of pseudo-precocious puberty (mainly breast development), a large pelvic mass with high plasma oestradiol and urinary oestrogen levels, and low gonadotrophins. In the adult, periods become irregular, with breakthrough bleeding from a hyperplastic 'cystic' endometrium. After the menopause, the presentation is likely to be with postmenopausal bleeding. Thecomas (benign tumours of thecal cell origin), which are about one-third as common, also secrete oestrogens; they tend to occur in an older age group, and are almost always benign. Arrhenoblastomas are benign sex-cord stromal tumours which contain Sertoli and/or Leydig cells. They are only about one-fifth as common as granulosa cell tumours, and usually present in young women with virilisation due to secretion of large amounts of testosterone and/or androstenedione. Germ cell tumours (gonadoblastomas) almost always arise in abnormal gonads, particularly in individuals with a Y chromosome. Such a gonad is potentially dangerous and, in such individuals, both gonads should be removed. An interesting category of virilising tumour is the Krukenberg tumour, where a secondary tumour metastasising to the ovary stimulates the stroma to produce androgens. In occasional women with virilising tumours presenting in pregnancy it appears that human chorionic gonadotrophin has stimulated a previously-inactive ovarian tumour. Teratomas of the ovary occasionally produce chorionic gonadotrophin, leading to precocious sexual development, and occasionally to virilisation. A teratoma occasionally contains thyroid tissue, and may present with thyrotoxicosis! Finally, ovarian carcinoid tumours have been described, as have tumours that secrete ACTH and cause Cushing's syndrome. There are indeed a very wide range of possible endocrine manifestations of ovarian tumours.

The Gonads and Cancer

Breast cancer

The breast is an oestrogen target-organ, and some breast cancers (about one-third) are dependent upon oestrogens for their continuing growth. Such tumours are often the better-differentiated ones, which therefore tend to have the best prognosis anyway. Castration and adrenalectomy, or hypophysectomy, have now largely been replaced by the use of anti-oestrogens (e.g. tamoxifen) in the management of oestrogen-dependent breast cancer. Responsive tumours possess oestrogen receptors, and respond to oestrogens in ways similar to normal target tissue.

Endometrial cancer

Endometrial cancers are stimulated by oestrogens and are often highly responsive to progestogens such as medroxyprogesterone acetate. The risk of inducing endometrial cancer as a consequence of giving unopposed oestrogens has probably been exaggerated, but an occult cancer may certainly be stimulated into growth.

Prostatic cancer

A situation exists similar to that with breast cancer.

The better-differentiated prostatic cancers possess androgen receptors and are, at least partially, androgen-dependent. The use of anti-androgens such as cyproterone acetate, or inhibition of gonadotrophin secretion by a long-acting GnRH analogue are at least of temporary palliative value in such cases, and have largely replaced the use of castration for treatment.

6

The Parathyroid Glands and Common Disorders of Bone

The parathyroid glands produce parathyroid hormone which is one of the factors involved in the precise regulation of the serum calcium. A primary increase in parathyroid hormone secretion will lead to hypercalcaemia while a decrease causes hypocalcaemia. However, many non-parathyroid disorders can affect the serum calcium so that it is best to consider parathyroid disorders as part of the wider study of causes of a high or low serum calcium.

ANATOMY

There are normally four parathyroids, lying immediately behind the upper and lower poles of the thyroid gland. Variations in situation and occasionally number of the glands are not unusual. The glands consist of two cell types — the chief cell and oxyphil cell — though different functions have not been ascribed to them (Fig. 6.1).

The parathyroid glands produce a polypeptide hormone — parathyroid hormone (PTH). It contains 84 amino acids and, like many hormones, is derived from a precursor molecule (pro-PTH) and this in turn from a larger molecular weight pre-pro-PTH. Within the serum both the intact hormone and a variety of hormone fragments exist. Only those fragments with at least the first 32 amino acids present retain biological activity. Much of the PTH present in the blood as measured by most radioimmunoassays is likely to be biologically inactive (Fig. 6.2).

One of the main target organs of parathyroid hormone is bone, which is also the main store of calcium within the body. Far from being an inert organ, bone is constantly being remodelled by the action of osteoclasts and osteoblasts. Osteoclasts are multinucleated giant cells (Fig. 6.3), rich in lysozomal enzymes and acid phosphatase, which actively resorb bone.

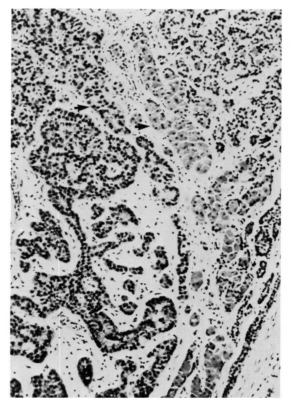

Fig. 6.1 *Normal parathyroid (H&E × 160). Islands of chief cells (small dark cells) and collections of oxyphil cells (larger paler cells) — separated by fibro-fatty tissue.*

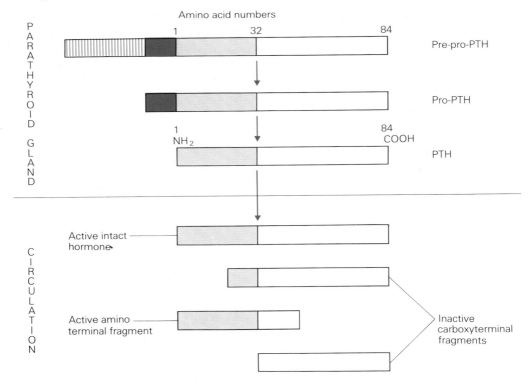

Fig. 6.2 *Diagrammatic representation of PTH biosynthesis and metabolism after entry into the circulation. The complete 1–32 amino terminal sequence is necessary for biological activity.*

Osteoblasts (Fig. 6.4), rich in the enzyme alkaline phosphatase, produce collagen fibres which are an essential part of the osteoid tissue on to which hydroxyapatite crystals are deposited to produce bone. Bone formation and bone resorption are closely interrelated and, under most situations, the two are equal.

PHYSIOLOGY

For normal body functions it is necessary to maintain the serum calcium within very closely controlled limits. Calcium is essential for muscle contraction, nerve conduction, blood clotting, gland secretory activity and many other vital processes. The normal serum calcium ranges between 2.20 and 2.60 mmol/l and calcium exists within the blood in three forms. The most important is ionised calcium, which is the physiologically active form and which constitutes almost one-half of the total calcium. Calcium binds to a number of proteins, particularly to albumin, and the protein-bound fraction amounts to almost half of the total calcium under normal circumstances; the small remaining fraction is complexed to substances such as phosphate and citrate. Because of the difficulties in measuring ionised calcium, virtually all routine measurements are of total calcium. This usually closely mirrors the ionised calcium, provided there is no great change in the serum proteins. However, in hypoproteinaemic states, e.g. malignancy, liver disease, nephrotic syndrome, the amount of protein-bound calcium is

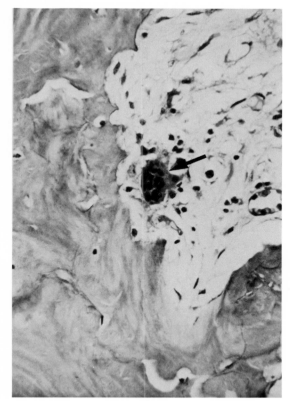

Fig. 6.3 *Multinucleated osteoclast within a resorption lacuna in a case of Paget's disease (H&E × 400).*

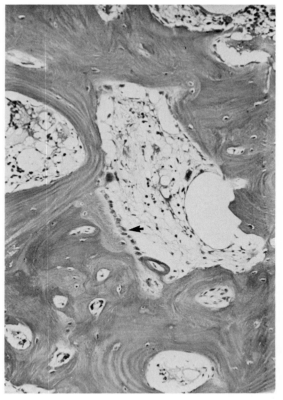

Fig. 6.4 *Osteoblastic bone formation (H&E × 252). A row of plump osteoblasts lining pale-staining osteoid seam.*

reduced; there is thus a fall in total calcium while the ionised calcium remains normal. Conversely, a condition leading to an increased total serum protein will increase the protein-bound calcium and hence the total serum calcium. Increased concentrations of serum proteins occur in dehydration and after prolonged venous stasis. Serum globulins bind calcium to a significant, but lesser, degree than albumin but this may be sufficient to increase the total serum calcium in those conditions associated with marked increases in the serum globulins, e.g. myeloma. Various protein correction formulae have been devised, but all are inadequate. It should be remembered that the normal range for serum calcium is appropriate only for samples with normal serum proteins. Under these circum-

stances total serum calcium closely correlates with ionised calcium. In any situation where there is a marked change in the proteins, this correlation disappears and the total serum calcium may be an inappropriate measure of the normality or abnormality of ionised calcium.

The serum calcium is maintained by regulating the amount of calcium absorbed by the gut or reabsorbed by the kidney and by the net flux of calcium in or out of bone. Figure 6.5 indicates the magnitude of the changes of calcium occurring daily at these three sites. Although the bones contain a large store of calcium (99% of the total body calcium of 25 mol), it is now thought that the rapid minute-to-minute control of serum calcium is dependent on small changes in the

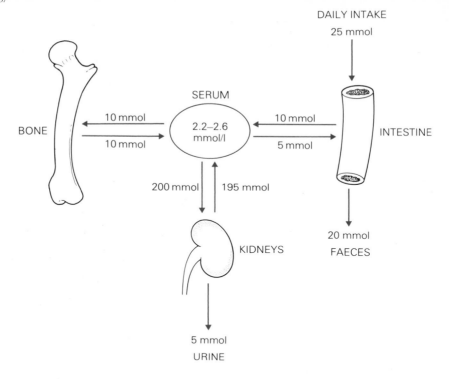

Fig. 6.5 *Schematic representation of calcium balance.*

renal calcium resorptive mechanism, where by far the largest daily turnover in calcium occurs.

A variety of factors influence calcium metabolism but two are of paramount importance – parathyroid hormone and vitamin D. Parathyroid hormone has its main actions on the kidney and bone where, in each site, it leads to an increase in calcium passing back into the circulation and hence to a rise in serum calcium. The secretion of parathyroid hormone is inversely related to serum calcium so that a fall in serum calcium to low levels leads to increased hormone secretion. Conversely, an abnormally high serum calcium suppresses hormone secretion.

Vitamin D Metabolism

Vitamin D is formed in the skin by the action of sunlight on the precursor 7-dehydrocholesterol. The vitamin formed is cholecalciferol (vitamin D_3). Vitamin D is also ingested in our diet either as ergocalciferol (vitamin D_2) or cholecalciferol. Under normal circumstances the vast majority of vitamin D originates from skin production and only a minor component comes from the diet. Both forms of vitamin D are relatively inactive and are initially converted in the liver to 25-hydroxy vitamin D and subsequently in the kidney to the active form of the vitamin: 1,25-dihydroxy vitamin D (1,25-di(OH)-vit D). In addition, the kidney can also produce 24,25-dihydroxy vitamin D (24,25-di(OH)-vit D) an inactive compound (Fig. 6.6). The relative amounts of these two compounds of renal origin vary depending on the physiological stimuli acting at the time. 1,25-di(OH)-vit D has a marked effect on the small intestine, increasing calcium absorption. Although a lack of vitamin D causes rickets or osteomalacia, it has

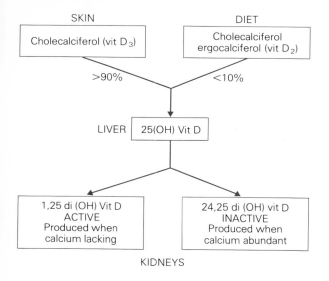

Fig. 6.6 *Schematic representation of vitamin D metabolism.*

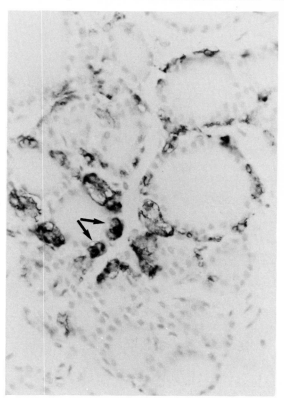

Fig. 6.7 *Parafollicular cells immunostained for calcitonin (× 500). Rat thyroid has been used, as normal human thyroid tissue contains very few parafollicular cells.*

not been possible to demonstrate a direct effect of vitamin D on bone formation. The vitamin acts by helping to provide the appropriate minerals for bone formation. Vitamin D compounds do, however, cause release of calcium from bone and, when present in excessive amounts, can cause severe hypercalcaemia. Basically, 1,25-di(OH)-vit D is produced in preference to 24,25-di(OH)-vit D in situations of calcium lack. There is also a further relationship between parathyroid hormone and the vitamin D metabolites, in that parathyroid hormone itself stimulates 1,25-di(OH)-vit D production. In this way, both act to ensure an effective response to hypocalcaemia or hypercalcaemia.

So far no mention has been made of calcitonin, a hormone produced by the parafollicular cells of the thyroid gland (Fig. 6.7). Although calcitonin has hypocalcaemic actions in animals, it does not seem to play a major role in the control of calcium homeostasis in humans. Calcitonin in humans only has a significant hypocalcaemic effect in those with a pathological increase in bone turnover, e.g. Paget's disease.

Tests of Parathyroid Function

Obviously, the most appropriate test of parathyroid

function would be the accurate measurement of parathyroid hormone concentrations. Although parathyroid hormone can be measured by radioimmunoassay, this assay is available only in a limited number of laboratories. Many assays have difficulties in accurately measuring normal or low hormone concentrations. Most assays measure both active and inactive fragments of PTH. The latter tends to accumulate in renal failure.

Before the availability of parathyroid hormone assays, and because of the continuing unavailability of an assay service in some areas, a number of indirect tests of parathyroid hormone activity have been devised. Many are based on the known phosphaturic actions of parathyroid hormone. Unfortunately none of

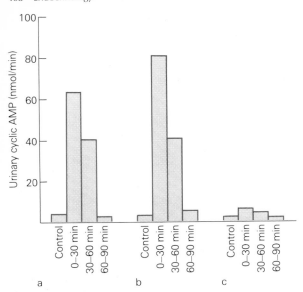

Fig. 6.8 *Cyclic AMP response to PTH in a normal* (a), *hypoparathyroid* (b), *and pseudohypoparathyroid patient* (c). *At 0 mins, PTH (200 units) is injected intravenously.*

Table 6.1

Symptoms of a Raised Serum Calcium

Tiredness and lethargy
Polyuria and nocturia
Thirst
Nausea and vomiting
Constipation
Mental confusion leading to coma when severe
Itching

in hospital inpatients. Symptoms of hypercalcaemia are very non-specific (Table 6.1) and often absent unless the hypercalcaemia is severe; rarely can a diagnosis of hypercalcaemia be confidently made on the basis of the clinical history and examinaton. Consequently hypercalcaemia will only be regularly diagnosed if the serum calcium is routinely measured on all patients.

Although there are many causes of hypercalcaemia, malignancy and hyperparathyroidism account for the vast majority of cases seen in normal clinical practice: all other causes are rare (Table 6.2).

Table 6.2

Causes of Hypercalcaemia

Common causes
    Malignant states
    Primary hyperparathyroidism

Uncommon causes
    Thyrotoxicosis
    Sarcoidosis
    Vitamin D poisoning

Some rarer causes
    Acute renal failure
    Milk alkali syndrome
    Immobilisation
    Addison's disease

these tests is sufficiently reliable to justify their continuing use. Occasionally it is necessary to test whether a patient is able to respond normally to parathyroid hormone. This is particularly true in patients suspected of having pseudohypoparathyroidism, where there is thought to be a defect at or after the level of the parathyroid hormone receptor. In these circumstances, use is made of the fact that parathyroid hormone stimulates its receptors and leads to the production of cyclic adenosine monophosphate (cAMP). Following the injection of parathyroid hormone there is normally a prompt rise in plasma and urinary cAMP as a result of increased renal production of this compound (Fig. 6.8). Associated with this is a less reliable increase in urinary phosphate excretion. A failure of these changes suggests a peripheral resistance to hormone action.

HYPERCALCAEMIA

With the advent of biochemical screening hypercalcaemia has become a very frequent finding, especially

Hypercalcaemia of Malignancy

Many malignant states can be complicated by hypercalcaemia. The mechanism whereby the hypercalcae-

---

Table 6.3

Hypercalcaemia and Malignancy

Tumour sites most commonly associated with malignant hypercalcaemia
  Lung
  Breast
  Larynx and pharynx
  Renal tract
  Female genital tract

Prevalence of hypercalcaemia in various malignancies

Myeloma	33%
Lung	
Breast	
Larynx and pharynx	5%
Oesophagus	
Gastrointestinal tract	1%

---

mia is produced is at present ill understood. Hypercalcaemia is usually associated with disseminated disease, which is rarely at a curable stage. The most likely malignant causes of hypercalcaemia are shown in Table 6.3. This in part reflects their frequency as malignant conditions; however, some malignant states appear to cause hypercalcaemia more frequently than others, e.g. myeloma, and squamous cell compared with small cell carcinoma of the lung.

Presentation

Patients may present with symptoms of either the malignancy and/or hypercalcaemia. Almost invariably, signs or symptoms of the malignant state are present at the time the hypercalcaemia is recognised.

Diagnosis

This is usually straightforward, as evidence of the malignancy is apparent. When malignancy is suspected but not confirmed, knowledge of those tumours most likely to cause hypercalcaemia (Table 6.3) will guide investigations.

Because of the usual widespread nature of the malignant disease, various nonspecific abnormalities may be found in biochemical and haematological investigations. This may include a reduced albumin or elevated globulin, altered liver function tests, anaemia or an elevated ESR. All these changes are unusual in hyperparathyroidism. Serum parathyroid hormone concentrations are usually low.

Management

Malignancy is by far the commonest cause of severe hypercalcaemia. The nonspecific nature of the symptoms of hypercalcaemia, however, often leads to a failure to recognise the abnormality or to attribute them to the underlying malignancy or its treatment. If the underlying malignancy cannot be treated, serious consideration should be given to treating symptomatic hypercalcaemia, as this can lead to a marked improvement in the quality of life. If severe, initial treatment should be with large quantities of intravenous fluids, usually with added potassium because hypokalaemia often develops. This is usually sufficient to bring the calcium down to safe levels. Long-term treatment should be attempted using either oral steroids (40 mg prednisolone daily initially, reducing to the lowest effective dose) or with oral phosphate (0·5 g three or four times daily).

Hyperparathyroidism

Primary hyperparathyroidism is the second most common cause of hypercalcaemia in hospital inpatients, and the commonest cause in outpatients. Until recently, primary hyperparathyroidism was thought to

---

Table 6.4

Symptoms of Primary Hyperparathyroidism in Patients Requiring Surgical Treatment

---

Tiredness and muscle weakness	50%
Asymptomatic	25%
Headaches	18%
Constipation	20%
Renal stones	14%
Polyuria, nocturia, thirst	30%
Muscle aches	15%
Bone pain	1%

---

be predominantly a condition associated with bone disease or renal stones, but it is now recognised that these are less common manifestations of the disease. This change in presentation has resulted from the wider application of calcium measurements. Most patients are either asymptomatic or have mild, nonspecific symptoms (Table 6.4). In particular, mention should be made of the muscle weakness and tiredness that many patients notice which, combined with the fact that most patients are over the age of 65, is often attributed to 'old age'.

Presentation

Most cases today are brought to light as a consequence of the serum calcium being measured on a biochemical profile during the course of the investigation of a variety of nonspecific symptoms, or for completely unconnected reasons. Obviously any patient with renal stones should have serum calcium measured probably on at least three separate occasions; approximately 1–3% of patients with renal stones will be found to have hyperparathyroidism. Occasionally hyperparathyroidism may be a familial disorder with dominant inheritance. Three inherited conditions are recognised:

    a. Familial hyperparathyroidism where no other endocrine disorder occurs.

    b. Multiple endocrine neoplasia-type I (MEN-I), the association of hyperparathyroidism with pancreatic islet cell tumours and occasionally pituitary adenomata.

    c. Multiple endocrine neoplasia-type II (MEN-II), the association of hyperparathyroidism with phaeochromocytomata (often bilateral) and medullary thyroid carcinoma.

In all three situations, four-gland parathyroid hyperplasia is found more frequently than a parathyroid adenoma.

Diagnosis

The exclusion of other obvious causes of hypercalcaemia, combined with an elevated serum parathyroid hormone concentration in the presence of hypercalcaemia, is the basis of diagnosis. In less than 10% of patients, diagnostic radiological changes of hyperparathyroidism are seen, with the most common change

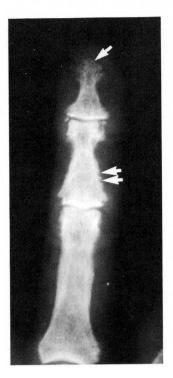

Fig. 6.9 *X-ray of hand in a patient with primary hyperparathyroidism showing subperiosteal erosions most marked in the middle phalanx and resorption of the terminal phalanx.*

being that of subperiosteal erosions that are seen best in radiographs of the hand (Fig. 6.9).

Management

The only effective treatment of primary hyperparathyroidism is parathyroidectomy. In about 90% of cases a single parathyroid adenoma is found. Occasionally there are multiple adenomata or hyperplasia of all four glands. Carcinoma is extremely rare.

The recognition of many mild asymptomatic cases of hyperparathyroidism, particularly in elderly patients, has led to a more conservative approach to management. Surgery is indicated in all cases with complications of the disease, and perhaps with young asymptomatic patients. More elderly patients with minor or no symptoms are now being followed conservatively in many centres. At present there is no safe, effective drug therapy for hyperparathyroidism.

Parathyroid surgery should only be performed by experienced parathyroid surgeons, in whose hands the incidence of unsuccessful surgery or postoperative complications is extremely low.

Secondary and Tertiary Hyperparathyroidism

Hypocalcaemia is a potent stimulus to parathyroid hormone secretion; any prolonged hypocalcaemic state will lead to secondary hyperparathyroidism with the development of high parathyroid hormone concentrations and hypertrophy of the parathyroid glands. Such states occur most commonly in vitamin D deficiency states (see p. 112) or in chronic renal failure. In chronic renal failure, hypocalcaemia occurs as a result of a failure to produce the active vitamin D metabolite 1,25-di(OH)-vit D in the kidney, and because of the high serum phosphate concentration. As a consequence, severe hypocalcaemia and bone disease can develop. The bone disease is usually a mixture of osteomalacia and of osteitis fibrosa caused by the parathyroid overactivity. More recently it has been recognised that aluminium toxicity may potentiate the serious bone disorder particularly in patients on long-term dialysis. The aluminium toxicity results from retention of small amounts of aluminium present in tap water used for dialysis or from absorption from the gut when aluminium hydroxide is used in an attempt to reduce high serum phosphate concentrations. Because of the impaired renal production of 1,25-di(OH)-vit D, renal osteodystrophy is resistant to treatment with calciferol but may be improved by using the synthetic vitamin D metabolites – 1α-hydroxy-cholecalciferol or 1,25-dihydroxycholecalciferol. These potent metabolites require careful monitoring because of their potential to cause hypercalcaemia. Some patients with renal osteodystrophy are hypercalcaemic. It is presumed that these patients developed the expected secondary parathyroid response to the hypocalcaemia of chronic renal failure. Subsequently, however, the enlarged parathyroids became autonomous and hypercalcaemia ensues. This state is called tertiary hyperparathyroidism. Such patients, as well as those with a normal or low calcium but with severe osteitis fibrosa unresponsive to vitamin D metabolites, require parathyroidectomy. At operation all four parathyroid glands are usually grossly enlarged. The traditional operation is to remove $3\frac{1}{2}$ glands but more recently there has been a tendency to remove all four glands and to reimplant fragments of one of the glands into the muscle of the forearm. This is in an attempt to prevent permanent hypoparathryoidism and also to provide easy access to the remaining parathyroid tissue should it become overactive again.

Other Causes of Hypercalcaemia

As shown in Table 6.2 there are a number of other causes of hypercalcaemia but they are relatively unusual in clinical practice. Vitamin D poisoning is a complication that may be encountered in patients treated with large doses of calciferol (doses usually of 100 000 units or more) or any patient treated with the normal pharamacological doses of the more active metabolites. Patients on such treatment require life-long monitoring to prevent such occurrences. Large doses of vitamin D (i.e. 100 000 units/day) are basically only needed in the treatment of hypoparathyroidism. Vitamin D deficiency states rarely, if ever, require more than 1–2000 units daily. There is no justification for the use of large doses of vitamin D to treat chilblains, soft nails or osteoporosis. In thyrotoxicosis there is an increased bone turnover and, in a small number of severely hyperthyroid patients, hypercalcaemia develops which is corrected by control of the hyperthyroid state. If, on treating the thyrotoxicosis, hypercalcaemia persists then concomitant hyperparathyroidism should be considered. Hypercalcaemia is an uncommon complication of sarcoidosis but appears to be due to an unexplained overproduction of 1,25-di(OH)-vit D in these patients. Other evidence of sarcoidosis is usually present but occasionally may be absent. Such patients should be expected to have low PTH concentrations and the hypercalcaemia is rapidly corrected by corticosteroid therapy – an unusual finding in hyperparathyroidism.

HYPOCALCAEMIA

The causes of hypocalcaemia are listed in Table 6.5. As mentioned earlier, because of the binding of calcium to serum proteins, the total serum calcium may be low in hypoproteinaemic states while the ionised calcium is normal. Hypocalcaemia can occur in both acute and chronic renal failure and this has been discussed previously.

Table 6.5

Causes of Hypocalcaemia

Common causes
    Spurious due to associated low serum proteins
    Renal failure
    Vitamin D deficiency states

Uncommon causes
    Hypoparathyroidism
    Hypomagnesaemia
    Acute pancreatitis

Some rarer causes
    Pseudohypoparathyroidism
    Aminoglycoside therapy

Vitamin D Deficiency States

Hypocalcaemia can occur in any vitamin D deficiency state but because of the secondary parathyroid response this is seldom severe and not infrequently the serum calcium may be around the lower limits of normal. A deficiency of vitamin D leads to the development of rickets in children and osteomalacia in adults. In addition to vitamin D deficiency, there are rarer causes of rickets and osteomalacia (Table 6.6).

Pathophysiology

In Britain, vitamin D deficiency occurs most commonly in Asians, where subnormal 25(OH)D concentrations

Table 6.6

Causes of Rickets and Osteomalacia

Vitamin D deficiency:
    Asians
    Elderly
    Gastrointestinal disease
    Liver disease
Anticonvulsant therapy
Vitamin D dependent rickets
Vitamin D resistant rickets
Tumoral rickets
Hypophosphatasia

are found in a large proportion of subjects. Usually this is without any clinical or biochemical consequences but, at times of greater vitamin D requirements, clinical disease may appear. It is for this reason that clinical disease is seen mainly in neonates, young children, adolescents and pregnant mothers. The exact reason for the high prevalence of vitamin D deficiency in Asians is unclear. It is unlikely that the deficiency is due to a simple dietary lack of vitamin D, and present evidence would not support a reduced production in the skin as a consequence of skin pigmentation. Although the precise mechanism is unclear, vitamin D deficiency is noted particularly in vegetarians with a high chapatti intake.

Recently increasing evidence has been obtained that suggests that vitamin D deficiency may be common in elderly people of all nationalities in Britain. The cause of this is presumably due to the inability of such people to get out into the sunlight; it is seen especially in the elderly housebound. Other causes of vitamin D deficiency include gastrointestinal disease, particularly malabsorptive disorders and liver disease.

Presentation

Presentation of vitamin D deficiency is varied and tends to differ depending on the age of the patient.

Neonates: Babies of Asian mothers tend to be smaller at birth and are more prone to hypocalcaemia and to have convulsions. The increased risk of these problems can be eliminated by supplementing the mother with vitamin D during pregnancy. Occasionally frank rickets may be present at birth.

Children and adolescents: Impaired growth may occur in the absence of bone pain. Bone pain is, however, the rule in these children and it commonly occurs in the knees. The pain is persistent and aggravated by exercise. Deformities are common and include bow legs and knock knees (Fig. 6.10). In the presence of severe hypocalcaemia, epileptic fits may occur.

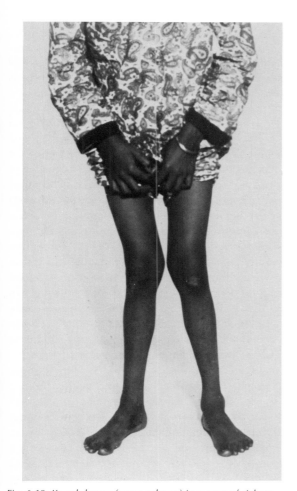

Fig. 6.10 *Knock knees (genu valgum) in a case of rickets.*

Adults: Bone pain is the main symptom in adults. It is often a widespread pain affecting many parts of the body. It may be severe enough to interfere with sleep. A waddling gait may develop which is particularly striking in pregnant patients.

The elderly: The exact clinical significance of suboptimal vitamin D concentrations in the elderly is at present unclear. Whether it plays any role in the aetiology of wrist and hip fractures and in the development of osteoporosis is controversial. Because osteomalacia is so readily treated it should always be considered in patients presenting with the above conditions.

Diagnosis

The prerequisite of diagnosis is a high index of suspicion. Many Asians are at risk of vitamin D deficiency, and conditions such as 'rheumatism', 'growing pains' and epilepsy should never be diagnosed until rickets or osteomalacia have been excluded. Clinical examination is often unhelpful unless the disease is severe. In children important signs include swelling over the metaphysis of the long bones especially the wrist, expansion of the costochondral junctions to produce the 'rickety rosary' and the deformities of bone mentioned earlier. In adults deformity of bone is not present unless the disease is complicated by fractures.

Biochemical changes include a serum calcium which is typically mildly reduced though occasionally very low. The serum phosphate is reduced and the alkaline phosphatase increased, due to an increase in the enzyme originating from the bone. This latter change is particularly difficult to interpret in young children and adolescents when rapid growth normally causes the serum alkaline phosphatase to be elevated compared with values seen in adults.

Radiological changes are frequently but not invariably present. In children they should be sought at the metaphysis of growing long bones, an x-ray of the wrists or knees being usually sufficient (Fig. 6.11a). In adults the classical radiological changes are appearance of pseudofractures (also called Looser's zones or Milkman's fractures). These are most commonly seen in the rami of the pelvis, femoral necks, scapulae and ribs (Fig. 6.11b).

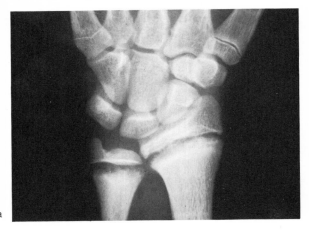

a

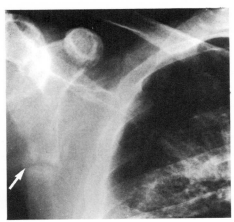

b

Fig. 6.11 (a) *Radiological changes of rickets showing widening and irregularity of epiphysis and* (b) *osteomalacia with a Looser's zone or pseudofracture in the wing of the scapula.*

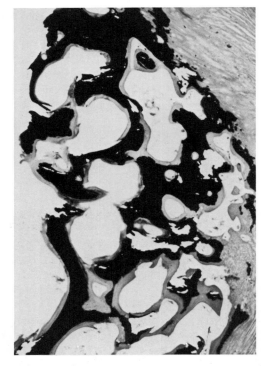

Fig. 6.12 *Histological changes of osteomalacia (undecalcified section, von Kossa stain × 252). Broad osteoid seams cover all trabecula (stained black).*

Bone biopsy will show the histological changes of osteomalacia with increased width of the osteoid seams (Fig. 6.12) but is rarely indicated.

Treatment

The vast majority of cases of vitamin D deficiency can be anticipated and hence ideally prevented. Routine vitamin D supplements should be given to all Asian expectant mothers to protect both mother and child. All Asian neonates and young children should receive multivitamin supplements and a case could be made for supplementing all Asian adolescents around the period of their growth spurt. All patients with malabsorption or those who for any reason cannot get out into the open air for long periods of time should be considered as potential candidates for developing vitamin D deficiency. A single tablet of calcium with vitamin D BPC given daily provides 500 units of vitamin D, which is an adequate prophylactic dose that is entirely safe and does not require biochemical monitoring. Babies can be treated with multivitamin drops so as to provide 400 units/day of vitamin D.

Established rickets and osteomalacia can be treated with similar preparations, but doses of 1000–2000 units per day are preferred. Except in very exceptional circumstances, use of large doses of vitamin D or active metabolites of vitamin D is never indicated as they carry with their use the definite risk of hypercalcaemia.

RARER FORMS OF RICKETS AND OSTEOMALACIA

Vitamin D-dependent Rickets

This form of rickets, which is inherited as an autosomal recessive condition, has clinical and biochemical features identical to vitamin D deficiency rickets, but fails to heal on small doses of vitamin D. Larger doses of around 50 000 units/day cause complete healing. The condition is thought to be due to a deficiency of the 1α-hydroxylase enzyme in the kidney that converts 25(OH)D to 1,25-di(OH)-vit D.

Vitamin D-resistant Rickets or Hypophosphataemic Rickets

This condition has a number of features that are quite different from the previous causes of rickets. The serum calcium is always normal and the main biochemical feature is marked hypophosphataemia.

A basic defect in phosphate transport is the likely underlying problem rather than a disorder of vitamin D metabolism. Various forms of the disease are seen. Both a dominant and a sex-linked form have been described. In some, multiple defects of proximal renal tubular function (Fanconi's syndrome) may be present. An identical condition (tumoral rickets) is also seen in the presence of slow-growing tumours particularly of the skin and muscle. Removal of the tumour cures the rickets. Treatment of vitamin D-resistant rickets is difficult and complete healing does not occur even with massive doses of vitamin D. The best results are probably obtained with combined phosphate and vitamin D treatment.

Hypoparathyroidism

Causes

Hypoparathyroidism is most commonly seen following neck surgery as either a transient or permanent phenomenon. It occurs as a permanent condition after thyroidectomy in about 1% of cases. It is also rare following the removal of a single parathyroid adenoma but the risk increases if more parathyroid tissue has to be resected. Major neck resections for carcinoma of the larynx have a high incidence of hypoparathyroidism.

Rarely, hypoparathyroidism may be idiopathic. Some such patients have evidence of autoimmune disease and may have other autoimmune endocrine deficiency disorders, e.g. hypothyroidism, hypoadrenalism. These patients are prone to severe, widespread monilial infections.

Presentation

In the postoperative situation, symptoms of hypoparathyroidism usually develop 2–4 days after surgery, although there may occasionally be a long period between surgery and presentation. Idiopathic hypoparathyroidism may occur at any age. Symptoms include paraesthesiae, especially around the mouth and in the extremities, and tetany. In tetany, painful muscular contractions occur. A typical feature is the development of the 'main d'accoucheur', when there is flexion of the metacarpophalangeal joints and extension of the interphalangeal joints (Fig. 6. 13). When severe, hypocalcaemia may cause epileptic convulsions.

Diagnosis

A generalised hyperexcitability of muscle may be associated with positive Chvostek's and Trousseau's

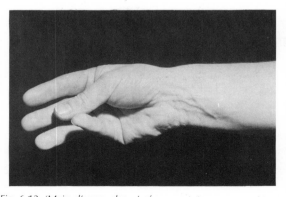

Fig. 6.13 'Main d'accoucheur' of severe tetany.

signs. Chvostek's sign is a contraction of the facial muscles when the facial nerve is gently tapped in the area overlying the temporo-mandibular joint. Although typically seen in hypocalcaemic states, it is occasionally positive in normal subjects. Trousseau's sign is elicited by inflating a sphygmomanometer cuff to just above systolic blood pressure. If positive, the hands contract into the *main d'accoucheur* position (Fig. 6.13). This can be a painful procedure for the patient and should not be performed excessively.

The serum calcium is low while the serum phosphorus is elevated. The serum alkaline phosphatase is normal.

Management

Following parathyroidectomy, transient mild hypocalcaemia is usually seen; this is often asymptomatic and does not require treatment. If it is more severe, treatment with intravenous calcium may be necessary. More persistent hypocalcaemia will need treatment with vitamin D. Calciferol, 100 000 units daily, is given together with intravenous calcium. Careful monitoring of the serum calcium is required, and gradually the intravenous calcium is reduced and stopped as the serum calcium rises. If hypoparathyroidism is permanent, long-term calciferol will be required. To be certain of this, attempts should be made to reduce the dose gradually to check whether hypocalcaemia recurs. Once stabilised, patients must remain under constant supervision. Most patients can be controlled on 100 000 units of calciferol daily. The serum calcium should be checked every 3–6 months for the rest of the patient's life. Patients should be advised to report immediately if symptoms of hypercalcaemia develop.

Pseudohypoparathyroidism

This is a rare inherited condition associated with peripheral resistance to parathyroid hormone. The biochemical changes of hypoparathyroidism are present despite high concentrations of circulating PTH. Resistance to injected PTH can be shown by a failure to increase cyclic AMP and phosphate excretion in the urine (Fig. 6.8). More recent studies have shown that the PTH receptor in the kidney is normal but that there is a defective post-receptor mechanism. Clinically such patients tend to be short and obese with a moon facies. The 4th and 5th metacarpals may be short. Mild mental retardation is common.

Hypomagnesaemia

Hypocalcaemia may be associated with hypomagnesaemia and may in fact be caused by it. The commonest causes of hypomagnesaemia are chronic alcoholism and gastrointestinal disorders. It may also be seen during long-term aminoglycoside therapy. In these circumstances the hypocalcaemia is extremely resistant to treatment until the hypomagnesaemia is corrected.

Acute Pancreatitis

Hypocalcaemia is a not infrequent complication of acute pancreatitis, although the exact explanation is unclear. Severe hypocalcaemia is indicative of severe pancreatitis and a poorer prognosis. Very occasionally hyperparathyroidism is associated with pancreatitis. The elevated serum calcium may fall to normal levels transiently after an episode of pancreatitis and can easily be missed unless the serum calcium is checked after complete recovery.

COMMON DISORDERS OF BONE

Osteoporosis

Pathophysiology

Bone is constantly being remodelled, and bone formation and resorption are closely linked. Bone density remains constant during adult life until the fifth decade when it begins to decline. This is more marked in females, especially as they become postmenopausal. The reason for the decline in bone mass is a slight excess of bone resorption over bone formation. Such changes occur in everybody as they age and cannot be considered to be abnormal. The process, however, seems to be exaggerated in some individuals. The loss of bone particularly affects trabecular bone and hence the consequences of these changes are predominantly seen in the vertebral bodies and ends of the long bones, e.g. neck of femur and distal radius, where trabecular bone is proportionately greater.

Presentation

The inevitable loss of bone with age means that the changes of osteoporosis are often found coincidentally during the investigation of other conditions. The commonest symptoms are related to fractures of the distal radius, femoral neck and vertebrae. The latter typically cause acute, severe back pain which settles in 4 to 6 weeks. Repeated fractures result in an increased spinal kyphosis and loss of height. Chronic back pain is much more difficult to evaluate, and the discovery of osteoporosis does not necessarily indicate an aetiological role.

Diagnosis

To produce a convincing change on standard radiographs, at least 20–25% of skeletal calcium has to be lost. More sensitive radiological techniques involve careful measurements of the cortical thickness of the metacarpals. A yet more sensitive method involves the measurement of the amount of gamma irradiation which passes through a bone – absorption bone densitometry. There are no biochemical changes in osteoporosis. Histological examination reveals normal bone reduced in amount (Fig. 6.14).

Management

Ideally, osteoporosis should be prevented before it produces fractures. It now seems clear that the administration of oestrogens at or shortly after the menopause delays or prevents the loss of calcium. Oestrogen therapy has to be given cyclically, combined with progestogens, for many years. Unfortunately no technique has yet been discovered for predicting those patients who will have an exaggerated loss of bone and hence be at greatest risk of subsequent complications. At the present time it is not common practice to offer oestrogens to asymptomatic postmenopausal women.

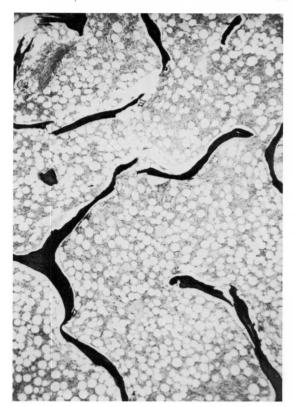

Fig. 6.14 *Osteoporosis of lumbar vertebral body showing marked atrophy of bone trabeculae (HVG × 160). This and other histological illustrations in this chapter by courtesy of Professor E. L. Jones.*

In established osteoporosis the goal of treatment is to increase bone density, and many treatments have been advocated. Considerable confusion about the efficacy of these treatments exists, mainly due to the difficulty of measuring small changes in bone density. Commonly used regimes include calcium supplements, vitamin D and oestrogens. Because of the claims that osteomalacia may be a common factor in cases of long bone fracture in the elderly, this condition should always be sought.

Paget's Disease

Pathophysiology

Epidemiological studies have shown this to be a common condition, occurring in about 4% of subjects over the age of 50. The incidence increases with age and shows a marked geographical variation. It is common in subjects from Western Europe and North America. In Britain, it is most prevalent in the north-west of England. Within the nucleus of osteoclasts affected by Paget's disease are to be found inclusion bodies resembling viral particles. This has raised the possibility that Paget's disease is the result of a slow virus infection.

Presentation

Most people with Paget's disease are completely asymptomatic and the condition is found accidentally. A small proportion of patients develop symptoms, of which the commonest is localised bone pain. Expansion

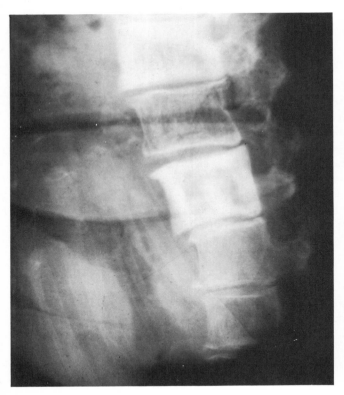
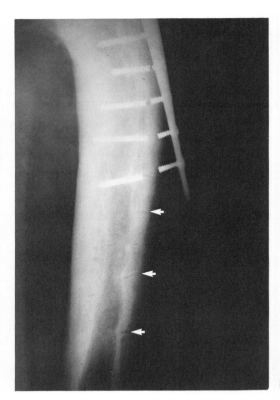

a b

Fig. 6.15 *(a) Paget's disease of lumbar vertebra – showing abnormal texture and enlargement of bone. (b) Femur affected by Paget's. Note thickened cortex with multiple 'fissure fractures' in the deformed bone. Screws inserted after previous hip fracture have been snapped by the progressive deformity.*

of bone may lead to deformities and to nerve compression especially of the auditory nerve. Fractures are more common in Pagetic bone, especially when it is deformed. Fortunately the development of an osteogenic sarcoma is an extremely rare complication; it presents with rapid swelling and increased pain in the affected bone.

Diagnosis

The radiological features of Paget's disease are usually diagnostic; bone shows an abnormal trabecular pattern, with a mixture of increased and decreased bone density, associated with expansion of the affected bone (Fig. 6.15). The disease may affect one or multiple bones. Commonly-affected bones are the vertebrae, pelvis, skull, femur, tibia and clavicle. The serum alkaline phosphatase is usually elevated due to an increase in the isoenzyme originating in the bone. Isotope bone scans show increased uptake, which can mistakenly be diagnosed as secondary deposits.

Treatment

The main indication for treatment is pain. Asymptomatic patients do not require treatment. Pain should initially be managed with simple analgesics; only when these fail should specific treatment be considered. Two treatments are available: calcitonin and diphosphonate drugs. Calcitonin has to be administered by subcutaneous injections. A dose of 100 units of salmon calcitonin daily is usually given for initially 6 to 9 months. After injections, patients may feel transiently flushed or nauseated. Of patients who respond, about one-third subsequently relapse despite continuation of therapy.

Sodium etidronate, a diphosphonate, is an oral treatment for Paget's disease; a dose of 5 mg/kg is given daily for 6 months. On cessation of treatment a prolonged remission may occur, though most patients relapse and require further courses of treatment. Intermittent therapy is used to prevent the development of osteomalacia, which was once a common consequence when higher doses were used.

Fractures should be treated by conventional means. Osteogenic sarcomas arising within Pagetic bone carry a very bad prognosis despite surgical or chemotherapeutic treatment.

7

Endocrine Effects of Tumours

ECTOPIC HUMORAL SYNDROMES

Introduction

Even though a clinically recognisable case was first described in 1896 it was not until twenty years ago that the syndrome of ectopic ACTH production was recognised. A patient was described who had Cushing's syndrome due to bilateral adrenal hyperplasia. The ACTH driving the adrenal glands, however, was produced not by the pituitary gland but by a bronchogenic carcinoma. Lung (bronchial) tissue is not normally the site of significant ACTH production, hence the use of the word ectopic to describe its secretion.

Although bronchogenic carcinoma, particularly of the small or oat-cell variety, remains the commonest tumour associated with ectopic humoral syndromes, there are now a number of other tumours which have been shown to produce ectopic hormones. It has been suggested that, for some tumours, hormone production is the rule rather than the exception. Confusion has sometimes arisen, with regard to the definition of ectopic production, when tumours produce more than one hormone, one of which is not ectopic while the other is. Certain islet cell tumours of the pancreas produce both insulin (non-ectopic) and ACTH (ectopic), and thus what was initially thought to be a simple concept has become a little blurred in some cases. The present discussion is confined to true ectopic production of hormones.

The tumours to be discussed have certain features in common; it is apparent that the cell types involved in ectopic hormone production are derived from a common embryological source, even though they may be widely scattered within the body. They are all neuroendocrine cells which are derived from the primitive neural crest. Tumour cells produced from these precursor cells have characteristic histochemical reactions which distinguish them. They are capable of the uptake of amine precursors and subsequent decarboxylation of these. The initials of amine precursor uptake and decarboxylation, APUD, have been used to describe such cells, and the tumours have often been called apudomas on the basis of these histochemical reactions. The final products of such cells are rarely amines, however; secretion of simple amino-acid chains (polypeptides) are more commonly seen. Occasionally, glycoprotein hormones are produced. It has been suggested that the primitive stem cell has the DNA capacity to develop into a number of different organs but most genetic material is normally repressed during development. The phenomenon of derepression, allowing the ability to make simple endocrine substances, is thought to occur in apudomas.

Table 7.1 outlines the various hormones produced by tumours. There is not always a clinical syndrome associated with hormone production, and some tumours are capable of producing a variety of hormones. On occasion more than one hormone is produced by the same tumour in the same patient. As already indicated small cell carcinoma of the bronchus is the commonest tumour associated with ectopic hormone production, and Fig. 7.1 shows the typical histology of such a tumour.

For the physician it is the clinical manifestation of hormone excess which may first indicate the presence of a tumour, but the true incidence of such syndromes is not known with certainty. Studies on the biosynthesis of ACTH by small cell tumours suggest that over 90% of these can synthesise ACTH. The advent of sensitive radioimmunoassay techniques for measuring polypep-

Table 7.1

Hormones Produced by Tumours

Ectopically-produced hormones	Clinical hormone syndromes	Associated neoplasms
ACTH	Cushing's syndrome	Small cell bronchogenic ca, ca thymus, ca pancreatic islet
LPH (β-lipotrophin)	?Hyperpigmentation in ectopic ACTH syndrome	Bronchial carcinoid, medullary ca thyroid
HCG (human chorionic gonadotrophin)	Gynaecomastia, precocious puberty	Small cell bronchogenic ca, hepatoblastoma
AVP (arginine vasopressin)	Inappropriate ADH (AVP) syndrome	Small cell bronchogenic ca, ca pancreas (rare)
TGF (transforming growth factor)	Hypercalcaemia	Squamous cell bronchogenic ca, kidney ca, ovary ca
OAF (osteoclast activating factor)	Hypercalcaemia	Myeloma
NSILA	Hypoglycaemia	Fibrosarcoma
Erythropoeitin	Erythrocytosis	Uterine fibromyoma, cerebellar haemangioblastoma
Chorionic somato-mammotropin or HPL (human placental lactogen)	None	Small cell bronchogenic ca
GH (growth hormone)	?Hypertrophic pulmonary osteoarthropathy	Small cell bronchogenic ca
GH releasing factor	Acromegaly	Bronchial carcinoid, pancreatic islet carcinoid
HCG (TSH-like)	Hyperthyroidism	Choriocarcinoma
Prolactin	Galactorrhoea	Hypernephroma
Hypophosphataemia-producing substance	Hypophosphataemia – osteomalacia	Mesenchymal tumour
Enteroglucagon	Gastrointestinal abnormalities and symptoms	Renal tumour
CRF (corticotrophin-releasing factor)	Cushing's syndrome	Bronchial carcinoid, prostatic ca
Calcitonin	None	Small cell bronchogenic ca, medullary ca, thyroid and breast ca
VIP (vasoactive intestinal polypeptide)	Watery diarrhoea	Small cell bronchogenic ca

tide hormones has uncovered the fact that many tumours can and do produce polypeptides which are biologically inactive, and it is now clear that the clinical syndromes represent only the tip of the iceberg in terms of the secretory capacity of tumour cells.

The Clinical Syndromes

The ectopic ACTH syndrome

As indicated above, this was the first of the ectopic humoral syndromes to be described and has been the most widely reported of all. It is most commonly associated with small cell carcinoma of the bronchus which accounts for some 60% of cases. Ten per cent are associated with thymic or pancreatic tumours, and about 4% with bronchial carcinoids. The bronchial carcinoid tumour represents a particular category of cells of the APUD series.

Most students and clinicians will be aware of the classic clinical presentation of Cushing's syndrome, with centripetal obesity, plethora and abdominal striae (see Chapter 4). Such features are rarely seen with ectopic ACTH production, particularly if it is associated with a malignant tumour. Most of these patients are

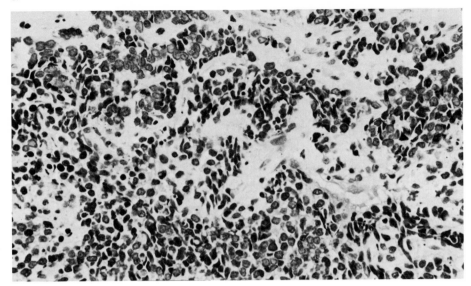

Fig. 7.1 *Small (oat) cell carcinoma of bronchus. Infiltrating cells have irregular nuclei varying in hyperchromicity (slide by courtesy of Dr M. A. McIntyre, Dept. of Pathology, Western General Hospital, Edinburgh).*

cachectic, and it seems that the overwhelming effects of the carcinoma together with the rapid downhill course of the disease give little time for the glucocorticoid effects of cortisol to be manifest. A small group of patients with more benign tumours such as bronchial carcinoids secreting ACTH, represent the exception to this rule in that the more typical features of Cushing's syndrome are then observed.

Most patients with ectopic ACTH production are male, reflecting the higher incidence of smoking, still thought to be the main aetiological factor for bronchogenic carcinoma. Pigmentation is common and is due to the melanocyte stimulating activity of ACTH and related peptides which may also be secreted by the tumour. Diabetes is often present, and a hypokalaemic alkalosis, usually with hypertension, is the rule. These latter features are thought to be related to excess mineralocorticoid activity and possibly represent the effect of excessive production of cortisol and deoxycorticosterone by the zona fasciculata under the influence of ACTH (Fig. 7.2), the effect being to retain

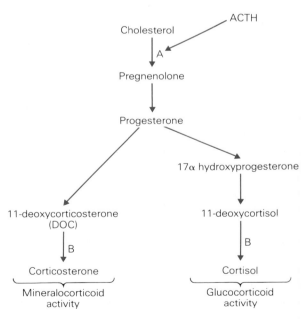

Fig. 7.2 *Effects of ACTH on steroidogenesis within the adrenal cortex. Aminoglutethimide acts at site A to reduce all steroid production while metyrapone inhibits 11-β-hydroxylation at site B preventing the formation of cortisol and corticosterone.*

Table 7.2

Characteristic Clinical and Biochemical Features of Pituitary-driven Cushing's Disease and Ectopic ACTH Production

Feature	Pituitary	Ectopic
Sex	F > M	M > F
Age	< 50	> 50
Anorexia	no	yes
Weight loss	no	yes
Marked pigmentation	rare	yes
'Cushingoid'	yes	not usually
Low serum K (< 3.0 mmol/l)	no	yes
Marked elevation of ACTH (> 300 ng/l)	no	yes
Suppressibility of ACTH and cortisol with high-dose dexamethasone (8 mg daily)	yes	no
Exaggerated ACTH and 11-deoxycortisol response to the 11β-hydroxylase inhibitor metyrapone	yes	no

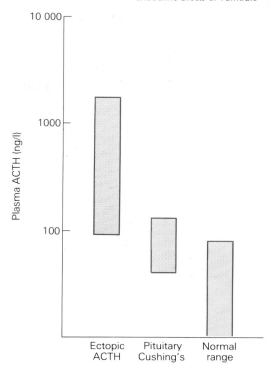

Fig. 7.3 Plasma ACTH levels in ectopic ACTH dependent Cushing's syndrome are generally much higher than that seen in the pituitary-driven form of the syndrome.

sodium at the expense of potassium, hence giving rise to a volume mediated hypertension. The dissimilarities between pituitary-driven Cushing's disease and the ectopic form can be seen in Table 7.2.

The biochemical hallmark of this condition is, of course, excess cortisol production and there is a lack of the normal circadian variation such that plasma cortisol levels remain high in the evening. Plasma levels of ACTH measured by radioimmunoassay are high, usually being much higher than those seen in the pituitary-driven form of Cushing's disease (Fig. 7.3). There remains no doubt that the ACTH is secreted by the tumour cell in that it has been detected in tumour tissue at post-mortem and can be shown to be synthesised by cultured tumour cells.

In the formation of ACTH, much larger biologically inactive precursor molecules are produced, variously known as pro-ACTH (pro-opiocortin) or 'big' ACTH. During enzymatic cleavage of these precursor molecules, other peptides – β-lipotropin and β-endorphin – are produced, and these have also been detected in excessive amounts in both plasma and tumour tissue from such patients. High levels of big ACTH (where ACTH has not been cleared from the

N-terminus of the pro-opiocortin molecule) are rarely seen in pituitary-driven Cushing's disease, and can thus help to differentiate the two conditions. The clinical presentation is such, however, that confusion is unlikely in most patients, particularly those with malignant disease. The most commonly employed method to distinguish the two conditions is based on the observation that ACTH production in pituitary-driven Cushing's disease is not entirely autonomous and can be suppressed by the administration of a large dose of dexamethasone (8 mg/day), which acts via the normal negative feedback loop to inhibit ACTH production. Suppression of ACTH by dexamethasone is rarely seen in ectopic production.

The prognosis for patients with bronchogenic carcinoma in general is poor. Surgery for small cell tumours has been shown to be ineffective, and radiotherapy is usually reserved for local symptoms.

Chemotherapy can sometimes improve survival, and can ameliorate the clinical syndrome. In such cases, the secretion of peptide hormones may provide markers for the recurrence of the disease process.

If metabolic effects of excess glucocorticoid or mineralocorticoid activity are troublesome, then the administration of certain drugs which inhibit steroidogenesis may be helpful. Aminoglutethimide inhibits the early step of conversion of cholesterol to pregnenolone (site A, Fig. 7.2) and metyrapone prevents the final hydroxylation step in the production of cortisol (site B, Fig. 7.2). Metyrapone is better tolerated than aminoglutethimide, which frequently produces skin rashes and somnolence.

Hypercalcaemia

The differential diagnosis of hypercalcaemia is discussed in Chapter 6. However, the commonest cause of a raised serum calcium among hospitalised patients is malignancy, probably accounting for about 60% of cases. The most common malignancies associated with hypercalcaemia are carcinomas of the bronchus, breast and renal tract, together with myeloma (see Table 6.3). The mechanism for hypercalcaemia is reasonably clear when bony metastases are apparent, probably relating to simple bone destruction with release of calcium into the circulation. Small bony metastases can be difficult to detect even after radionuclide bone scanning, but there are patients in whom hypercalcaemia does not appear to be related to direct bone destruction. In these cases it is likely that there are circulating factors which can affect serum calcium. There are clear examples of patients in whom hypercalcaemia resolved when the primary tumour alone was removed, but what these factors are remains uncertain. It is probable that there is more than one hypercalcaemic agent associated with malignancy and in some patients a parathyroid hormone-like substance has been isolated, particularly in association with a squamous cell carcinoma of the bronchus and with hypernephroma. Even in these patients, however, many of the biochemical features seen in primary hyperparathyroidism, e.g. increased calcium absorption from the gut and increased urinary phosphate excretion, are not seen and it is thus not clear how important ectopic parathyroid hormone production is

in mediating hypercalcaemia in such patients. Currently available radioimmunoassays for parathyroid hormone are not reliable enough to give a definitive answer to this question.

Several peptides have now been discovered, produced by tumours, that are capable of activating osteoclasts. These have been termed 'transforming growth factors' (TGF), and an alpha and a beta type have been identified. They are at least 100 times more potent than PTH in activating bone reabsorption. Using genetic engineering techniques, *E. coli* bacteria have been made to synthesise TGF.

The observation that indomethacin and similar drugs that inhibit the production of prostaglandins also lower serum calcium in some cases of malignant hypercalcaemia has led to the suggestion that tumours may release substances that give rise to local prostaglandin production and bone destruction. Prostaglandins belong to a group of substances (discussed later with reference to the carcinoid syndrome) which may represent the final common mediators of many hormonal actions throughout the body (see Chapter 1). As they are normally destroyed during passage through the lungs, it seems unlikely that prostaglandins themselves could be circulating factors in mediating hypercalcaemia.

Hypercalcaemia is sometimes associated with haematological malignancies, particularly myeloma, and it is known that circulating substances may mediate osteoclast activation in these conditions as well as in some solid tumours. A lymphokine seems to be the most likely candidate for this; the current terminology is 'lymphotoxin' in view of the observation that it is also toxic to lymphocytes.

A not uncommon problem in clinical practice is the differentiation of patients with malignant hypercalcaemia from those with primary hyperpaparathyroidism. This can be difficult, particularly if no other clinical or radiological clues are available. The response to glucocorticoid can be helpful as a discriminator. For reasons which are not clear, after the administration of hydrocortisone (40 mg three times a day for ten days) the hypercalcaemia associated with malignancy *usually* improves whereas that associated with primary hyperparathyroidism remains unaltered.

The clinical features associated with malignancy are no different from those of hypercalcaemia of any cause, and they include anorexia, thirst, polyuria, constipation and mental disturbance. If it is asymptomatic, hypercalcaemia may not require specific therapy; with symptomatic hypercalcaemia, serum calcium levels should be lowered initially by rehydration. Some physicians use large volumes of intravenous saline together with diuretics which enhance calcium excretion (frusemide or bumetanide). This regime necessitates very careful management of fluid balance. Thiazide diuretics tend to increase serum calcium and should be avoided. If this mode of therapy proves ineffective, glucocorticoids can be used, together with calcitonin (a hypocalcaemic hormone that blocks resorption and is normally produced by the C cells of the thyroid gland) or phosphate therapy. The risk of the latter is in precipitating calcium in tissues, but this may not be important if the aim is mainly to palliate a terminal condition. The cytotoxic agent mithramycin has also been shown to be very effective in lowering serum calcium and has been used to good effect. Treatment directed at the specific tumour involved would obviously be desirable, but this is rarely successful in practice.

The syndrome of inappropriate antidiuretic hormone secretion (SIADH)

Under normal circumstances, fluid intake is associated with a transient fall in plasma osmolality; this is sensed by the osmoreceptors in the hypothalamus, and antidiuretic hormone (vasopressin) secretion is reduced. If fluid is withheld, plasma osmolality rises and antidiuretic hormone secretion is stimulated. The relationship of plasma osmolality to antidiuretic hormone levels in blood is a linear one (Fig. 7.4). Hyponatraemia seen in the setting of malignancy is most often associated with a small cell carcinoma of the bronchus and results from the autonomous secretion of antidiuretic hormone by the tumour. The fall in osmolality of plasma which occurs when fluids are ingested by patients with this syndrome does not reduce the secretion of antidiuretic hormone, and thus a dilutional hyponatraemia results. Under these conditions the normal relationship between plasma osmolality and circulating levels of antidiuretic hormone is abolished (Fig. 7.4). It should be noted that large amounts of antidiuretic hormone are not required to produce severe hyponatraemia which, in this situation, is

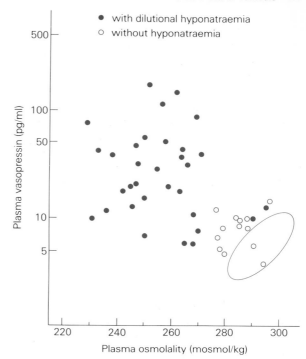

Fig. 7.4 *Relationship of plasma levels of ADH (vasopressin) to plasma osmolality. The normal relationship is depicted by the ellipse. Patients with SIADH all lie outside this range (●) and patients with small cell bronchogenic tumours (○) without hyponatraemia often have inappropriately high radioimmunoassayable ADH.*

governed primarily by the amount of water drunk. As the low serum sodium results from dilution rather than depletion of sodium, blood urea levels tend to be low and the urinary excretion of sodium is normal.

It is of interest that, although the true role of antidiuretic hormone was not appreciated at the time, the first description of this syndrome in association with bronchogenic carcinoma was made as long ago as 1938. Until the advent of radioimmunoassay techniques for the measurement of antidiuretic hormone the definition of SIADH was based on a number of features:

1. Plasma osmolality and serum sodium are reduced.
2. Despite this, the concentration of urine is inappropriately high such that urine osmolality is usually in excess of that of plasma.

3. Urinary sodium remains normal in contradistinction to that seen in sodium-deplete states where urine sodium is often low.

This combination of biochemical abnormalities has been described in a number of clinical states (Table 7.3), not all of which have subsequently been shown to be associated with high levels of antidiuretic hormone in either blood or urine; thus, for strict accuracy, SIADH should nowadays include measurement of the antidiuretic hormone itself. Such assays, however, are not readily available and most clinicians are thus forced to rely on the above criteria.

If hyponatraemia is noted in a middle-aged patient (usually male) who is a smoker, then a diagnosis of

---

Table 7.3

Hyponatraemic States Which Have Been Attributed to SIADH

Intrathoracic conditions
  bronchogenic small cell tumour (rarely other tumours: see Table 7.1)
  tuberculosis
  bacterial pneumonia
  viral pneumonia
  Legionnaire's disease (hyponatraemia very common)
  post-mitral valvotomy
  lung abscess

CNS conditions
  head trauma
  viral and bacterial infections
  cerebral neoplasm
  Guillain–Barré syndrome
  subarachnoid haemorrhage

Drugs associated with hyponatraemia
  chlorpropamide
  vincristine
  clofibrate
  thiazide

Miscellaneous
  hypothyroidism
  hypopituitarism
  Addison's disease
  lymphoma
  acute intermittent porphyria
  fluid overload post-surgery

---

bronchogenic carcinoma should be strongly considered even if there are no radiological abnormalities. It is not unusual for hyponatraemia to precede chest x-ray abnormalities.

Clinical symptoms are unusual unless serum sodium is below 120 mmol/l, and are often precipitated by the ingestion of large volumes of fluid. It may well be that sudden large changes in osmolality may be more important in precipitating symptoms than the absolute level *per se*. Initial symptoms may be confusion and disorientation which can progress, as serum sodium falls, to convulsions and coma. As already indicated, the level of serum sodium is governed primarily by the fluid intake and in all patients serum sodium can be returned to normal by reducing the intake to between 500 and 1000 ml per day. There are occasional patients in whom this form of fluid restriction is difficult to enforce and the best treatment is then the use of demeclocycline 600–1200 mg/day. This drug prevents antidiuretic hormone from attaching to its receptor at the renal tubule and thus induces a state of nephrogenic diabetes insipidus, which counteracts the effects of too much antidiuretic hormone. Lithium carbonate, a drug commonly used in the treatment of manic-depressive psychosis, has a similar effect but is less predictable in its results and more toxic, and therefore is not to be recommended.

The administration of salt or mineralocorticoids is unnecessary and generally ineffective in the long-term treatment of hyponatraemia associated with antidiuretic hormone excess. In an emergency situation, however, where the patient is symptomatic, hypertonic saline can have a transient benefit when infused intravenously. Again, removal of the primary tumour or effective chemotherapy can correct the syndrome and measurement of circulating levels of antidiuretic hormone can provide a marker for recurrence of tumour.

When antidiuretic hormone is produced in the hypothalamus, it is produced in association with a presumed carrier protein, neurophysin. Both antidiuretic hormone and neurophysin have been detected in tumour tissue, again confirming the ectopic nature of hormone production in this condition. As is the case with ACTH, it is quite likely that many tumours produce ADH which is detectable in the radioimmunoassay (see Fig. 7.4), but it is uncertain whether this is always biologically active. However, approximately 40% of patients with small cell carcinoma are unable to excrete a water load, which suggests that inappropriate ADH secretion is much more frequent than is generally supposed.

It is of interest that patients who harbour tumours producing both ACTH and antidiuretic hormone do not necessarily have inappropriate antidiuresis since the hypokalaemia produced by ACTH excess induces a nephrogenic diabetes insipidus, thus counteracting the effects of the antidiuretic hormone.

Hypertrophic pulmonary osteoarthropathy

Finger-clubbing is common with bronchogenic neoplasms of all types. Hypertrophic pulmonary osteoarthropathy occurs particularly with squamous cell bronchogenic carcinomas. This condition affects the tibia, fibula, radius and ulna and is characterised by the laying down of new subperiosteal bone, thus giving rise to distal pain affecting the arms and legs. Some of the radiological features are similar to those seen in patients with acromegaly, and the suggestion has been made that growth hormone or a similar substance produced by the bronchogenic tumour might be responsible for this condition. Some patients with bronchogenic carcinoma do have elevated levels of growth hormone which fail to suppress normally following glucose loading. It is uncertain, however, whether this growth hormone is produced by the pituitary or is truly ectopic. Acromegaly has occurred in association with malignancy but, in such (extremely uncommon) cases, it is likely that a growth hormone releasing factor is produced by the tumour to stimulate the pituitary to release growth hormone. Such a factor has recently been purified from a pancreatic tumour (see Chapter 2).

Gynaecomastia

Gynaecomastia can occur as a normal phenomenon during puberty in males (see Chapter 5). When it occurs in middle age, however, the possibility of an underlying tumour should be considered. Certain drugs can give rise to gynaecomastia, particularly spironolactone and cimetidine, and possibly digoxin. Some 'endocrine' tumours, such as choriocarcinoma and testicular teratoma, secrete chorionic gonadotrophins which are not strictly ectopic. Hepatoma and squamous cell car-

cinoma of the bronchus can also secrete chorionic gonadotrophin which stimulates production of oestrogen and androgens by the interstitial cells of the testis. The oestrogen then produces gynaecomastia. The chemical structure of chorionic gonadotrophin consists of an alpha and a beta subunit which can be secreted separately by such tumours (see Fig. 1.6). These can be measured by radioimmunoassay. HCG alpha or beta subunits are secreted by many tumours and can be used as tumour markers. Treatment is directed at the primary tumour, but may also involve the use of an anti-oestrogen or, occasionally, mastectomy.

Hypoglycaemia

Hypoglycaemia is the natural consequence of excessive insulin secretion from a pancreatic islet cell tumour. This is not ectopic secretion as already indicated, but hypoglycaemia has been associated with a number of mesenchymal tumours, particularly retroperitoneal fibrosarcomata. It seems unlikely that true insulin is secreted by these tumours but other substances which have insulin-like activity are thought to be involved. It may be that these substances represent somatomedins but this is not at all clear and currently they are grouped together as Non-Suppressible Insulin-Like Activity (NSILA).

The symptoms of hypoglycaemia can be divided into those affecting the central nervous system, i.e. neuroglycopenia, and those peripheral hyperadrenergic effects related to the excessive production of catecholamines. The former consists of confusion and disorientation and even coma, while the latter includes palpitations, hunger and sweating. These symptoms can be intractable, often requiring the administration of large amounts of glucose. Some help can be obtained from the use of the hyperglycaemic agent, diazoxide.

Reference to Table 7.1 shows that there are a number of other hormones associated with tumours that have not been discussed in detail. Given our current knowledge, they represent even more rare problems than those discussed above but it may be that some peptides which are biologically inactive may be helpful as tumour markers. Thus discovery of ectopic hormone production may:

a. permit an early diagnosis of cancer to be made;

b. aid in the localisation of a non-radiologically demonstrable tumour;

c. aid in assessing the response to treatment.

Since many tumours produce biologically inactive hormones, it is clear that one cannot rely on clinical symptoms alone and that any screening procedure would have to depend upon radioimmunoassays. In the future it may be that groups of individuals at high risk, e.g. heavy smokers, might be screened for the presence of peptide hormones in blood in the hope that this might provide an earlier diagnosis and thus better long-term results from therapy.

CARCINOID SYNDROME

The term carcinoid was first introduced to describe intestinal tumours which, although looking somewhat like the more common adenocarcinoma, tended to be very slow growing and generally more benign. Carcinoid tumours can occur in many sites throughout the body and are examples of APUD cells as described above. Because of the embryological development of the neuroectodermal cells, carcinoid tumours are found in the gastrointestinal tract, pancreas and biliary tract, lungs (embryologically derived from the foregut), thymus and even the urogenital tract.

Carcinoid tumours can arise throughout the whole length of the gastrointestinal tract although the vast majority occur within the small bowel. The most common single site is the appendix, probably accounting for over half of all reported cases. Primary tumours are small, rarely greater than three centimetres in diameter. The tumour is submucosal and usually asymptomatic. Histologically the tumours are composed of small round cells having basophilic nuclei with abundant cytoplasm containing eosinophilic granules which often stain with silver salts, hence the name argentaffinoma; mitoses are rarely seen (Fig. 7.5). It is very difficult to classify these tumours as benign or malignant on the basis of histological appearances, and it seems that the size of the tumour is a good guide as to the risk of malignancy. Tumours smaller than 1 cm in

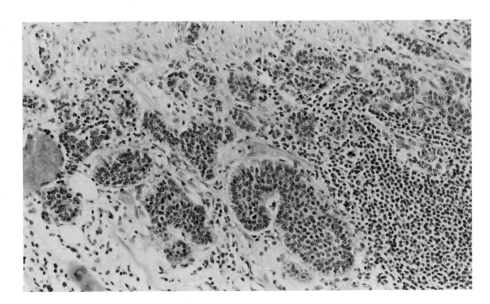

Fig. 7.5 *Ileal carcinoid: well circumscribed masses of cells showing peripheral pallisading and small regular nuclei (slide by courtesy of Dr M. A. McIntyre, Dept. of Pathology, Western General Hospital, Edinburgh).*

diameter rarely metastasise, while those greater than 2 cm often do. It is of interest that, although the carcinoid tumours arising in the appendix are by far the commonest, they are perhaps the least likely to give rise to metastases.

The bronchial carcinoid is in many respects similar to the small cell carcinoma and it may well be that these two conditions represent extremes of the same disease. Histologically, the bronchial carcinoid is similar to that seen in the gastrointestinal tract.

Although the incidence of carcinoid tumours may be of the order of 1% of all tumours, they remain mostly undetected during life — unless noted independently at appendicectomy — except when they metastasise. They would represent an uninteresting group of conditions if it were not for the observation that the tumour can, rarely, secrete vasoactive substances which result in characteristic symptoms and signs – the carcinoid syndrome.

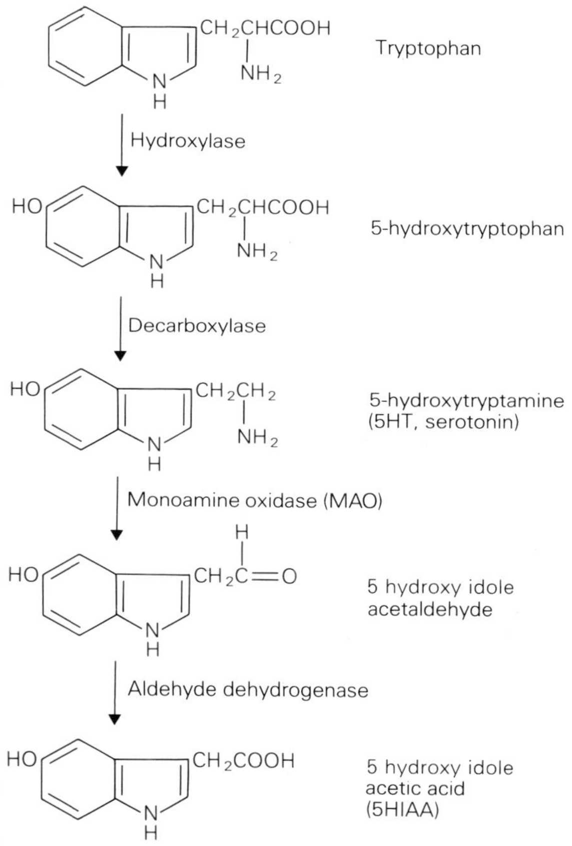

The full carcinoid syndrome is a complex involving facial flushing, diarrhoea, abdominal pain, cardiac failure due to peculiar valvular disorders of the right side of the heart and asthma. Less than 5% of patients with carcinoid tumour have the syndrome, which is thought to be caused by a variety of substances produced by such tumours. Serotonin (5-hydroxytryptamine) has been isolated from carcinoid tumours and is formed by hydroxylation of the amino acid tryptophan (Fig. 7.6). Tryptophan is derived from foods such as bananas and meats and, under normal circumstances, only about 2% of our dietary tryptophan is used to produce serotonin. The carcinoid tumour, or metastases from one, may metabolise up to 60% of the dietary intake in this manner.

Fig. 7.6 *Formation of 5-hydroxytryptamine (serotonin) from tryptophan, and breakdown to form 5HIAA.*

Clinical Presentation

Carcinoid syndrome is rare in children; it occurs most commonly between the ages of forty and sixty, equally in males and females. The commonest clinical features are: flushing in 95% of patients; diarrhoea in 85%; cardiac lesions with cardiac failure in 50%; and asthma in 22% (Fig. 7.7).

Flushing

Characteristically the patient develops an erythematous rash involving the head and neck area (similar to a blush), the attacks are paroxysmal (sometimes provoked by food or alcohol) and usually last for a few minutes only. The skin looks normal between attacks. Flushing is sometimes accompanied by a tachycardia but blood pressure rarely rises, unlike the paroxysms of hypertension usually seen in patients with a phaeochromocytoma, which is a condition also sometimes associated with flushing rather than the more usual pallor. Occasionally the flushing attacks can last longer and the skin retains a violaceous hue between attacks. Facial telangiectasia can then develop. When flushing is

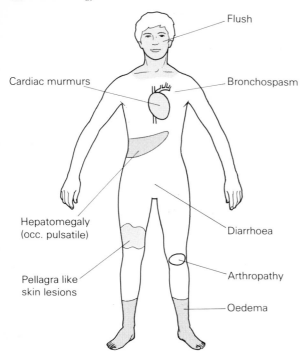

Flush

Cardiac murmurs

Bronchospasm

Hepatomegaly
(occ. pulsatile)

Diarrhoea

Pellagra like
skin lesions

Arthropathy

Oedema

Fig. 7.7 *Spectrum of clinical findings in the carcinoid syndrome.*

associated with a benign bronchial carcinoid tumour, the flush is often more prolonged and can last for days, sometimes involving the whole body. In this circumstance there are often associated symptoms of periorbital oedema, excessive lachrymation, diarrhoea and often hypotension with tachycardia.

Flushing attacks can be provoked by excessive exercise, anxiety or increasing emotion, and these triggers are thought to be related to catecholamine excess. As has already been mentioned, certain foods, e.g. cheese and alcohol, can precipitate attacks, or they may arise without any obvious precipitating cause.

Diarrhoea

Although diarrhoea is almost as common as flushing, the symptoms may not coexist in the same patient, thus suggesting a different cause. Hypermotility of the gut causes the diarrhoea, which is of variable amount and frequency.

Carcinoid heart disease

A unique constellation of cardiac features occurs in about 50% of patients with the carcinoid syndrome. A peculiar fibrosis develops on the luminal surface of the internal elastic lamina of the heart, causing whitish-yellow lesions that are covered by normal endothelium. These lesions involve the right side of the heart much more commonly than the left. The tricuspid and pulmonary valves are particularly affected, but not the pulmonary arteries. Probably because of the initial size of the respective valve rings, the functional effect is to produce a pulmonary stenosis and tricuspid incompetence. Similar lesions on the left side of the heart, affecting the mitral and aortic valves, are much rarer; they have been described in patients with congenital abnormal communications between the right and left side of the heart, as well as in patients with bronchial carcinoids where the presumed drainage of any vasoactive substances is into the left side of the circulation. The combination of pulmonary stenosis and tricuspid incompetence is particularly deleterious to the heart function, resulting in marked right-sided cardiac failure. The most reliable physical sign of cardiac involvement is the presence of a systolic murmur of pulmonary stenosis. The tricuspid murmur is usually less obvious, but 'v' waves can sometimes be seen in the jugular venous pulse and, if the liver is pulsatile, this is strong evidence for tricuspid incompetence. The progress of the cardiac lesions is variable, ranging from a rapid downhill course to a more prolonged, benign natural history.

Asthma

Patients commonly hyperventilate during attacks of flushing, but in about 20% of patients a true wheeze can be demonstrated that often coincides with flushing attacks.

Mechanism of the Carcinoid Syndrome

The aetiology of the various components of the carcinoid syndrome may be different. The observation that symptoms do not occur with GI carcinoid tumours unless there are liver metastases suggests either that the liver destroys a circulating factor or that a large bulk

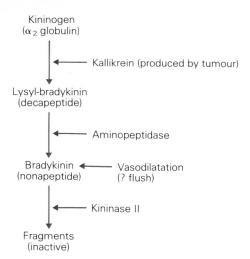

Fig. 7.8 *Formation of vasoactive bradykinin. Kallikrein is released from tumour tissue in response to catecholamine stimulation.*

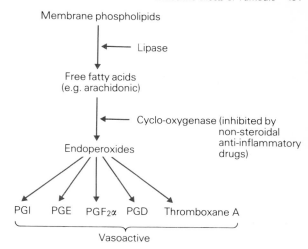

Fig. 7.9 *Prostaglandins are produced in cell membranes and those indicated have been shown to have powerful effects on blood vessels. It is possible that some of the symptoms of the carcinoid syndrome may be mediated via prostaglandin production.*

of tumour tissue is necessary before symptoms can occur. There seems good evidence that circulating factors are involved, and the first substance to be isolated from carcinoid tumours was serotonin. It is unlikely, however, that serotonin itself is solely responsible for the flush of the carcinoid syndrome and other vasoactive substances more recently detected in tumours are more likely candidates. Carcinoid tumours have been noted to produce kallikrein, an enzyme capable of producing bradykinin from an α_2-globulin substrate (Fig. 7.8). Bradykinin is an important vasodilating substance which could result in a flushing attack. It is thought likely that tumour kallikrein is released under the influence of catecholamines. Another group of vasoactive substances, the prostaglandins, which are fatty-acid derivatives, have also been implicated as a potential mechanism of flushing (Fig. 7.9).

Serotonin may well be the cause of the diarrhoea since serotonin antagonists such as methysergide will reduce the symptoms.

The cause of the carcinoid cardiac lesions is likewise uncertain but again a circulating factor, probably one which is inactivated during passage through the lungs, is probably involved. The fact that prostaglandins are destroyed during passage through the lungs makes it possible that these are implicated and serotonin may also be involved.

The relationship of asthmatic symptoms to tumour secretory products is unknown.

The Diagnosis of the Carcinoid Syndrome

As gastrointestinal carcinoid tumours do not produce the syndrome unless secondary spread (usually massive) to the liver is present, a radionuclide liver scan will commonly detect abnormalities in patients who have the syndrome. If the scan is positive in a patient with carcinoid syndrome then it is unnecessary to search for the primary tumour unless it is causing local symptoms or obstruction of the bowel. If scanning reveals no evidence of liver deposits, then a careful search for a primary lesion not draining into the hepatic circulation is indicated. These tumours are the bronchial and ovarian carcinoids, and they would require bronchoscopy or detailed gynaecological evaluation respectively.

More commonly, it is necessary to evaluate a patient presenting with a series of symptoms which may or may not be related to the carcinoid syndrome. If flush is a prominent feature in the history, this can often be provoked to simulate the disease and thus confirm the diagnosis. If a patient gives a history of alcohol-induced flushing, then this can be repeated under controlled conditions. The flush can almost always be precipitated by intravenous injection of noradrenaline or adrenaline, but this should be done under carefully controlled circumstances, with the initial dose of each being one microgram.

The biochemical hallmark of the disease is the increased urinary excretion of the 5-hydroxytryptamine metabolite, 5-hydroxy indole acetic acid (5HIAA). Care should be taken to exclude from the diet those foods, e.g. bananas, with a high tryptophan content. Drugs such as chlorpromazine, whose metabolites interfere with the assay of 5HIAA, should be discontinued before testing. All patients subsequently proven to have the carcinoid syndrome will have increased excretion of 5HIAA (normal range is usually 15–75 μmol/24h).

Treatment

When the carcinoid syndrome arises as a result of a bronchial or ovarian carcinoid draining directly into the systemic venous system, the surgical removal of a tumour may cure the syndrome. As gastrointestinal tumours will metastasise to the liver, a surgical cure would require resection of part of the liver. This is sometimes feasible due to the slow rate of growth of such tumours. Partial hepatectomy can dramatically reduce the symptoms of a carcinoid syndrome. It is rarely necessary to look for the primary tumour. Hepatic metastases have been ablated by the embolisation of the tumour by injection of foam to the hepatic artery. This is a relatively new technique but appears promising. The use of cytotoxic agents has been less successful, but combinations of cyclophosphamide, methotrexate or 5-fluorouracil and streptozotocin have been used with some success.

The ability of some carcinoid tumours to take up metaiodobenzylguanidine (MIBG) may be used therapeutically. This compound is a derivative of guanethidine, an adrenergic neurone blocker and, when labelled with radioactive iodine (^{131}I), can allow a visualisation of phaeochromocytomata and sometimes carcinoid tumours. This might be helpful not only in localisation of tumour metastases but, if the amount of radioactive iodine is great enough, it may be used therapeutically to destroy the metastases.

Pharmacologically, inhibitors of the formation of 5-hydroxytryptamine have been used, and these include α-methyldopa, parachlorophenylalanine and 5-fluorotryptophan. These have been used with some success. Methysergide, an antagonist of 5-hydroxytryptamine, may be of value in the treatment of diarrhoea. The use of kallikrein inhibitors such as trasylol has been disappointing, there being little effect on bradykinin production *in vivo*. Overall, therefore, drug therapy of this condition has been disappointing.

Ectopic Hormone Production

Carcinoid tumours have been associated with the production of ectopic hormones, including ACTH and insulin-like substances.

Prognosis

This is variable and depends to some extent on the site of the primary tumour. Where bronchial or ovarian tumours are detected, a complete cure can be expected as long as metastases have not occurred. When gastrointestinal tumours have metastasised to the liver, the likelihood of cure is remote; many such tumours are extremely slow-growing, however, and patients have survived for twenty years after the demonstration of metastatic deposits.

8

The Endocrine Pancreas

ANATOMY, DEVELOPMENT AND FUNCTION OF THE PANCREAS

The pancreas is a mixed exocrine and endocrine gland concerned with energy metabolism. It is situated behind the stomach, with its head in the loop of the duodenum and its body and tapering tail stretching retroperitoneally across the vertebral column to the left kidney, where it turns forwards into the lienorenal ligament to end in the hilum of the spleen (Fig. 8.1). The posterior surface of the head rests directly on the bile duct, the neck on the origin of the portal vein, and the body on the splenic vein which drains most of the

pancreas. Its arterial supply is via the coeliac and superior mesenteric arteries (Fig. 8.2), and a generous supply of nerve fibres enters with the pancreatic arteries. The pancreatic nerves originate in the coeliac and superior mesenteric plexuses and contain parasympathetic fibres from the vagi, sympathetic fibres from the greater and middle splanchnic nerves, and visceral afferent fibres.

The pancreas develops from two separate diverticula which arise opposite each other from the gut (Fig. 8.3a). The ventral bud arises close to the hepatic diverticulum and soon fuses into it so that the main pancreatic and bile ducts share a common entrance into the duodenum in the adult. Growth of the duodenal loop

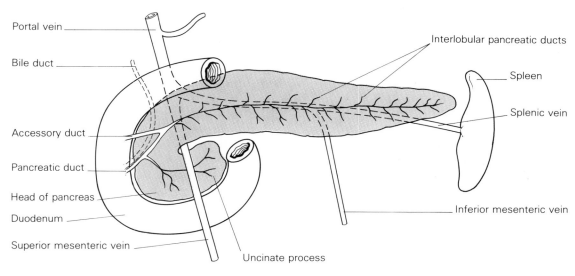

Fig. 8.1 *Anatomical relations of the pancreas.*

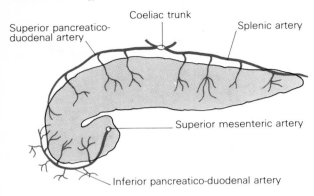

Fig. 8.2 *Pancreatic blood supply.*

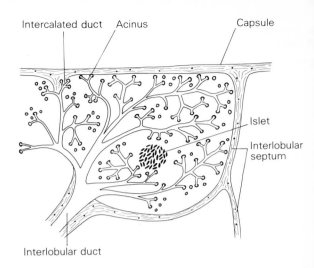

Fig. 8.4 *Structure of the pancreas: low power microscopy of pancreatic lobule.*

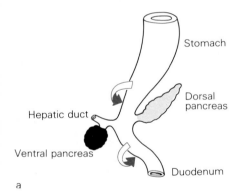

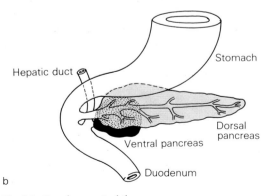

Fig. 8.3 *Development of the pancreas.*

causes the ventral pancreas and hepatic diverticulum to swing right round behind the gut until they impinge on the posterior and lower surface of the dorsal pancreas (Fig. 8.3b). The pancreatic primordia then fuse so that the ventral diverticulum ultimately forms the inferior part of the head and uncinate process and the dorsal diverticulum the remainder of the organ. The developing duct of the dorsal pancreas joins a tributary of the ventral duct so that the latter then becomes the terminal portion of the main duct. The terminal dorsal duct usually separates off as the accessory duct.

The pancreas is enclosed in a delicate fibrous capsule giving rise to septa which divide the gland into lobules. Microscopically, lobules are composed mainly of acini (i.e. serous cells producing pancreatic juice, grouped round a lumen) which drain into the pancreatic duct (Fig. 8.4). Thus, the great mass of the pancreas consists of exocrine tissue, endodermal in origin, whose main function is in relation to assimilation of energy and nutrients.

Sparsely scattered in the acinar tissue are tiny spherical masses of cells containing secretory granules but unconnected to ducts, the islets of Langerhans. These constitute the endocrine pancreas, which accounts for only 1–3% of the total pancreatic mass. Its cells originate from neuroectoderm and are of the

Table 8.1

*Distribution of Hormones and Amines Detected
in Endocrine and Nerve Cells*

	Endocrine cells			Nerve cells		
	Pancreas	Cell type	GI	Pancreas	GI	CNS
Polypeptide hormones						
Adrenocorticotrophic hormone	+		+	+	+	+
Bombesin	−		+	−	+	+
Cholecystokinin	+	A	+	+	+	+
Endorphin	+	A	+	+	+	+
Enkephalin	+	A	+	+	+	+
Enteroglucagon	+	A	+	−	−	+
Gastrin	−		+	+	+	+
Gastric inhibitory polypeptide	+	A	+	−	−	−
Glucagon	+	A	+	−	−	+
Insulin	+	B	−	−	−	+
Motilin	−		+	−	−	+
Neurotensin	−		+	−	−	+
Pancreatic polypeptide	+	PP	+	−	+	−
Secretin	−		+	−	−	−
Substance P	−		+	+	+	+
Somatostatin	+	D	+	+	+	+
Thyrotrophin releasing hormone	+		+	−	−	+
Vasoactive intestinal peptide	+		+	+	+	+
Amines						
Acetylcholine	−		−	+	+	+
Dopamine	−		+	+	+	+
Histamine	−		+	+	+	+
Noradrenaline	+	A,B,D	−	+	+	+
Serotonin	+	A,B	+	+	+	+

APUD type (p. 120, Chapter 7). They are part of a diffuse neuroendocrine system centred on the gastrointestinal tract which is concerned with the regulation of energy metabolism (Table 8.1). The roles of many of the hormones listed are poorly defined and most of the interrelationships between the various components of the system have still to be clarified, but its complexity suggests a capacity for fine tuning of energy metabolism.

THE ISLETS OF LANGERHANS: MICRO- AND ULTRASTRUCTURE

Within the larger system, the pancreatic islet is a functional unit composed of four main types of cells: A cells secreting mainly glucagon but also smaller amounts of at least five other hormones (Table 8.1), B cells secreting insulin, D cells secreting somatostatin, and PP cells secreting pancreatic polypeptide. In the adult, B cells constitute about 75%, A cells about 20%, and all other cell types 5%.

Human islets, especially the larger ones, are subdivided by bands of fascicular and connective tissue into subunits consisting of a central aggregation of B cells surrounded by a thin rim of varying numbers and types of non-B cells (Fig. 8.5). The islets contain, and are closely surrounded by, an unusually elaborate network of anastomosing capillaries, and the endothelial cells of the capillaries are fenestrated thus facilitating the rapid appearance of islet hormones in the circulation.

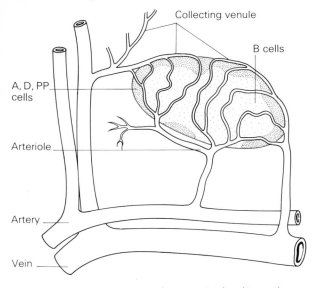

A, D, PP cells

Arteriole

Artery

Vein

Collecting venule

B cells

Fig. 8.5 *Microscopic structure of pancreatic islet of Langerhans.*

The cellular composition of the islets varies in different parts of the pancreas. In the tail, body and superior part of the head, A-cell-rich islets predominate, while in the middle and inferior part of the head PP-cell-rich islets are more numerous. Glucagon-rich islets belong to the part of the pancreas derived from the dorsal pancreatic bud which is vascularised by the coeliac trunk via the gastroduodenal, superior pancreatic duodenal and splenic arteries, and drained by the main dorsal and accessory exocrine ducts, while pancreatic polypeptide-rich islets are found in the part of the pancreas derived from the ventral pancreatic bud, vascularised by the superior mesenteric artery via the inferior pancreaticoduodenal artery and drained by the main ventral (or distal) exocrine duct.

Afferent arterioles enter the islet at gaps devoid of cells making it unlikely that intra-islet communication is mediated by blood-flow from non-B to B cells. Direct interaction between islet cells occurs via gap junctions. These are areas of common membrane of adjacent cells where ions and other small molecules can pass. They have been identified not only between B cells, but also between A and B or D cells, and have led to the concept of the islet as a functional syncytium.

Both sympathetic and parasympathetic nerve endings have been identified in close association with all four cell types.

Islet tissue increases in size throughout childhood and adolescence and reaches a constant of about 1 g in adult life. In the first three years of life there is an increase in the number of islets from about 300 000 at birth to about 1 000 000. Thereafter, the increase in weight of islet tissue is due to an increase in the size of individual islets to three or four times their size at birth. The capacity of the B cell to replicate appears to be finite and limited. Premature maturation of B cells may result in premature ageing with reduced insulinogenic reserve in later life.

INSULIN

The molecular weight of insulin is about 6000. The complete chemical structure of insulin was elucidated in 1955 by Sanger working in Cambridge, and was the first protein to have its structure determined. It is composed of two chains of amino acid residues: an A chain of 21 amino acids and a B chain of 30 amino acids, joined by two disulphide bridges. A third disulphide bridge connects one part of the A chain with another part of the same chain. It is formed from a larger, 80% less active, single-chain precursor, proinsulin (molecular weight 9000), which is then folded so that the disulphide bridges are formed correctly (Fig. 8.6). An even larger insulin precursor of about 11 500 daltons, pre-proinsulin, is synthesised initially on the rough endoplasmic reticulum. This has a very short half-life and is cleaved almost immediately within the cysternae of the endoplasmic reticulum to yield proinsulin.

Because the amino acid composition of insulin of different species varies relatively little, the antiserum directed against insulin of one species usually cross-reacts with insulin of other species. Moreover, since proinsulin of different species contains the same antigenic determinants in the insulin portion of the molecule, anti-insulin serum generally cross-reacts with heterologous proinsulin. In contrast, there are many species differences in the composition of C-peptide, so that C-peptide antisera are highly specific.

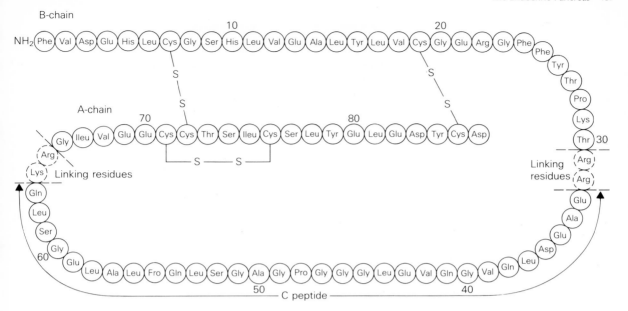

Fig. 8.6 *Structure of insulin.*

C-peptide is inert hormonally and metabolically. It has no receptors in the body, is not bound in the liver, and is excreted unchanged in the urine. Since C-peptide is secreted by the B cell in equimolar amounts with insulin, and because it is not metabolised and the assay is precise and specific, measurement of immunoreactive C-peptide in blood or urine is the best method of assessing the secretion of insulin by the pancreas *in vivo*.

To crystallise insulin it is necessary to add zinc or other metal ions, such as nickel, cobalt or cadmium. The three-dimensional structure of insulin crystals has been determined by Hodgkin and her colleagues at Oxford. Two atoms of zinc are usually found with six molecules of insulin in a spheroid unit: a hexamer. Dimers are also sometimes formed.

Insulin Biosynthesis, Storage and Release

Proinsulin is transported from the endoplasmic reticulum to the Golgi complex where it is packaged into granules (Fig. 8.7). Within the granules the connecting peptide is split off by proteolytic cleavage and insulin is complexed with zinc. The mature granules encased in smooth membranous sacs are released into the cytoplasm and become attached to the microtubular/microfilament system. When a stimulus for insulin secretion is received, a change occurs in the physical confirmation of the microtubules and the granules migrate to the cell surface where their contents are released by fusion of the membranous sac enclosing the insulin granule with the membrane of the B cell, followed by rupture and the release of equimolar amounts of insulin and C-peptide into the extracellular space (emiocytosis).

The adult human pancreas contains about 200 units (about 8 mg) of stored insulin. Microscopically, the number of B-cell granules is a good indication of the amount of insulin present in the pancreas and secretion of insulin is associated with degranulation of the B cell. Continuous stimulation of B cells by glucose results in an increase in the size of the nucleus and the rough endoplasmic reticulum, an increased number of ribosomes, and greater prominence of the Golgi apparatus. Synthesis and cleavage of proinsulin and storage of

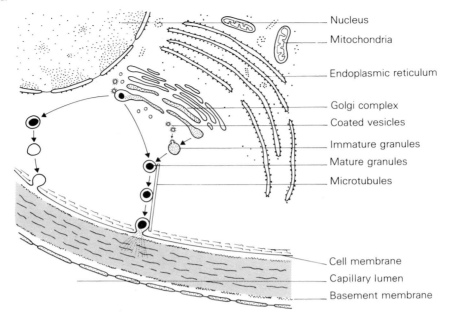

Nucleus
Mitochondria
Endoplasmic reticulum
Golgi complex
Coated vesicles
Immature granules
Mature granules
Microtubules
Cell membrane
Capillary lumen
Basement membrane

Fig. 8.7 *Ultrastructure of pancreatic B cell and the synthesis of insulin.*

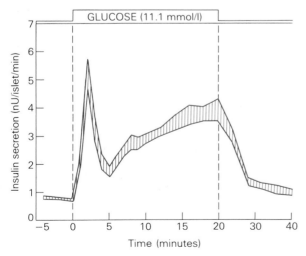

Fig. 8.8 *Biphasic secretion of insulin (mean ± SEM) by isolated, perifused rat islets in response to stimulation with 11.1 mM glucose.*

insulin are not directly coupled with release, and appear to be regulated separately.

Insulin is released in two situations, i.e. in the basal or steady state and in response to an external stimulus. The most important stimulus for insulin secretion is glucose.

The response to glucose can be studied *in vitro* using pancreatic islets separated from the exocrine tissue by digestion with collagenase. It is characteristically biphasic, the first phase being due to a small pool of insulin available for immediate discharge and the second to a large pool maintained by synthesis of insulin (Fig. 8.8).

In vivo there is an exponential relationship between the blood glucose concentration and the secretion of insulin into the pancreatic vein over a wide range of blood glucose concentration (Fig. 8.9). In normal subjects the concentration of immunoreactive insulin falls to an undetectable level in the peripheral blood when the blood glucose concentration is less than 2.2 mmol/l (40 mg/100 ml).

In clinical testing with oral glucose (Fig. 8.10) the first 30 minutes are dominated by the release of insulin from the small pool, insulin is released from the large pool during 30–90 minutes, and the rate of synthesis of

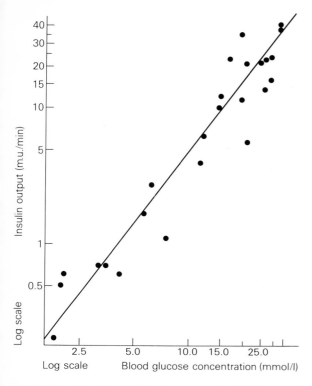

Fig. 8.9 *Secretion of insulin into the pancreatic vein of a normal dog in response to glucose.*

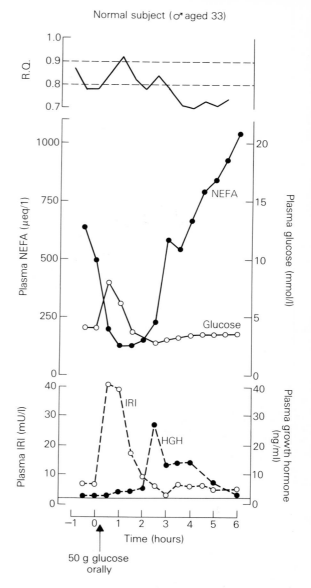

Fig. 8.10 *Changes in Respiratory Quotient and plasma concentration of glucose, non-esterified fatty acids, immunoreactive insulin and human growth hormone following ingestion of 50 g glucose by a normal, thin young man.*

insulin determines the secretion of insulin after 90 minutes.

When glucose is given by rapid intravenous injection the two phases of insulin secretion are more clearly separated. The rise in plasma insulin seen in the first 10 minutes represents insulin release from the small storage pool, whereas second-phase insulin release dominates the following 10–45 minutes (Fig. 8.11a).

The mechanism by which the plasma concentration of glucose regulates the secretion of insulin has not been precisely defined. The process is calcium-dependent, and two theories have been proposed: the glucoreceptor theory, suggesting that the molecule of glucose itself activates a stereospecific receptor on the B cell plasma membrane, and the metabolic theory, which suggests that in order to stimulate insulin release, glucose must be transported and metabolised in the pancreatic B cell and that changes in the concentration

of some intermediary metabolite initiate changes in insulin secretion. At the present time the balance of evidence favours the latter theory.

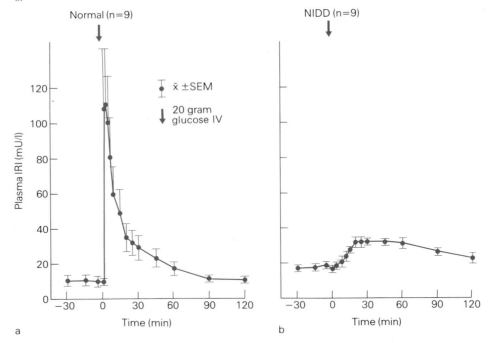

Fig. 8.11 *Concentration of plasma immunoreactive insulin following 20 g glucose intravenously in normal subjects and patients with NIDDM. Note the absence of first phase secretion of insulin in diabetic patients.*

Factors Directly Affecting the Secretion of Insulin

Substrates

During meals, substrates are the primary regulators of insulin secretion; carbohydrates, proteins and fats have all been shown to have a direct effect on the release of insulin by the B cell.

Glucose and fructose are the only important natural sugars regulating insulin secretion. Since fructose is largely converted to glucose during absorption and is a relatively weak stimulus, glucose is the dominant carbohydrate regulator.

Several amino acids increase insulin secretion. Arginine and leucine are the most potent in man. The mechanism of the amino-acid stimulation of insulin secretion appears to differ from glucose-stimulated secretion but glucose potentiates the secretion of insulin induced by some, but not all, amino acids. A substantial percentage of insulin secreted in response to a mixed meal is probably related to ingested protein.

Several fatty acids (octanoate, palmitate and oleate), and the ketone bodies 3-hydroxybutyrate and acetoacetate, are weak stimulators of insulin secretion and this is probably important in protecting the animal from developing severe ketoacidosis during prolonged fasting.

Pancreatic hormones

Glucagon enhances glucose-stimulated insulin secretion while somatostatin has the opposite effect.

Gastrointestinal hormones

A number of gastrointestinal hormones, including

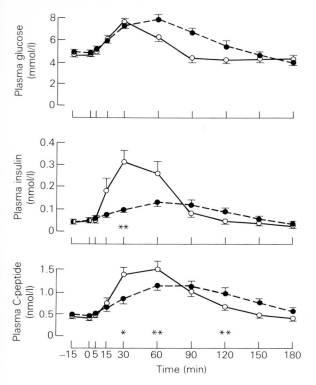

Fig. 8.12 *Mean (±SEM) concentration of plasma glucose, insulin and C-peptide in normal subjects after administration of an oral (O———O) and intravenous (●- - -●) glucose load designed to produce a similar plasma glucose concentration.*

gastrin, secretin, cholecystokinin (CCK), gastric-inhibitory polypeptide (GIP) and enteroglucagon, also enhance glucose- and amino-acid-stimulated insulin release but have little or no effect alone. GIP is probably the most important. This potentiation effect explains why the concentration of insulin in the peripheral

blood is greater after an oral than an intravenous glucose load designed to produce a similar plasma glucose concentration (Fig. 8.12).

α-Adrenoceptor agonists

Adrenaline, noradrenaline and clonidine are potent inhibitors of both basal insulin secretion and that evoked by a variety of secretagogues. Secretion of insulin is inhibited in patients with phaeochromocytoma and also possibly in normal subjects under stress.

Cholinergic agents

At physiological concentrations of glucose, cholinergic agents stimulate the release of insulin and this effect is abolished by atropine. Cholinergic activity mediated by vagal parasympathetic nerve fibres also enhances release of insulin (Table 8.2).

Sulphonylureas

Hypoglycaemic (e.g. tolbutamide and chlorpropamide, p. 171) and hyperglycaemic (e.g. diazoxide) sulphonylureas respectively stimulate and inhibit the release of insulin from the pancreatic B cell.

Other hormones

A number of other hormones can affect insulin secretion in response to a general metabolic need, such as exists in starvation (secretion of insulin reduced and delayed) and obesity and pregnancy (secretion of insulin increased). These include thyroid hormones, glucocorticoids, oestrogens, progesterone and somatomedins. Most of them antagonise the effects of insulin

Table 8.2

Summary of Autonomic Regulation of Islet Cells

Secretion of	Glucose	Acetylcholine	Noradrenaline
Insulin (B cell)	↑	↑	↓
Glucagon (A cell)	↓	↑	↑
Somatostatin (D cell)	–	↓	↑
Pancreatic polypeptide (PP cell)	–	↑	?

↑ = increase; ↓ = decrease; – = no significant primary effect.

in peripheral tissues and/or alter the insulin/glucagon ratio, thus producing a new steady state of increased secretion combined with decreased effectiveness of insulin.

Degradation of Insulin

Equimolar amounts of insulin and C-peptide, along with a small amount of proinsulin, are released by the pancreatic B cell into the portal vein. In the basal state (after a 16-hour fast) the secretion of insulin by the normal human adult pancreas is about 1 unit per hour. The half-life of insulin in blood is less than five minutes. Most tissues have the capacity to destroy insulin; the liver, kidney, pancreas and placenta are the most active and, in man, the liver removes 20–50% of insulin from the portal vein blood during a single passage. Two independent types of physiological degrading systems exist: tissue-based proteolysis by an insulin-specific protease, and the more important receptor-mediated degradation (see p. 145).

Actions of Insulin

Insulin has profound effects on carbohydrate, fat, protein and electrolyte metabolism (Table 8.3), which can be divided into anticatabolic and anabolic actions. The anticatabolic effects are important in the postabsorptive and fasting states whilst the anabolic actions come into play after meals (see below). In terms of total body fuel homeostasis, the prime targets are liver, fat and skeletal muscle although effects on other organs such as brain, small intestine, heart, lungs and leucocytes should not be ignored. The overall effects of insulin on the major metabolic organs are summarised in Fig. 8.13.

Liver

Insulin has many effects on liver metabolism. Glucose phosphorylation to glucose 6-phosphate, the first step in glucose utilisation, is enhanced through induction (increased synthesis) of glucokinase. Glycogen synthase is also activated, whilst phosphorylase is inhibited,

Table 8.3

Actions of Insulin

	Increase (anabolic effects)	Decrease (anticatabolic effects)
Carbohydrate metabolism	Glucose transport (muscle, adipose tissue) Glucose phosphorylation Glycogenesis Glycolysis Pyruvate dehydrogenase activity Pentose phosphate shunt	Gluconeogenesis Glycogenolysis
Lipid metabolism	Triglyceride synthesis Fatty acid synthesis (liver) Lipoprotein lipase (adipose tissue) activity	Lipolysis Lipoprotein lipase (muscle) Ketogenesis Fatty acid oxidation (liver)
Protein metabolism	Amino acid transport Protein synthesis	Protein degradation
Electrolytes	Cellular potassium uptake	

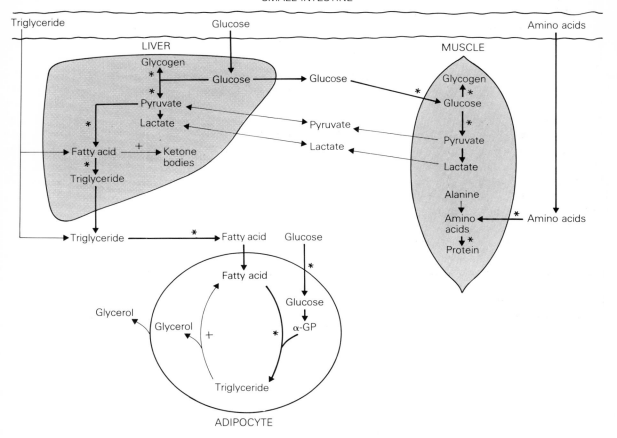

Fig. 8.13 *The overall effects of insulin on the major metabolic organs. * indicates pathways and processes stimulated by insulin. + indicates processes inhibited by insulin.*

resulting in net glycogen synthesis. Two further routes of glucose 6-phosphate metabolism, the pentose phosphate pathway and glycolysis, are also stimulated. At first sight, the latter would appear paradoxical, but this serves as a major route for conversion of excess glucose to fatty acid. The flow of substrate towards pyruvate is further enhanced by insulin inhibition of gluconeogenesis. Insulin also activates pyruvate dehydrogenase thus increasing the formation of acetyl CoA from pyruvate.

The first enzyme in fatty acid synthesis, acetyl CoA carboxylase, is also activated, yielding malonyl CoA and diverting acetyl CoA away from the citrate cycle and into fatty acid synthesis. Reducing equivalents required for fatty acid synthesis are provided by increased pentose phosphate pathway activity. *De novo* fatty acid synthesis is thus promoted and, after esterification with α-glycerophosphate, triglycerides are formed, which are secreted by the liver after conversion to very low density lipoproteins (VLDL). Again these latter processes may be stimulated by the action of insulin. Any already-formed long-chain fatty acids entering the liver will go through the same process in the presence of insulin. A further action on hepatic lipid metabolism is inhibition of ketogenesis. The probable mechanism involves an increase in malonyl CoA, which inhibits carnitine acyl transferase I, thereby preventing entry of acyl CoA into mitochondria from the cytosol and diverting the fatty acids into triglyceride and hence VLDL formation.

Hepatic protein metabolism is also influenced by insulin. Thus neutral amino-acid uptake pathways may be stimulated, as is protein synthesis. Finally hepatic potassium loss is also diminished by insulin.

Muscle

The prime action of insulin on carbohydrate metabolism in muscle is to stimulate glucose uptake. This is a relatively insensitive process which thus occurs most importantly when insulin levels are raised, probably through recruitment of glucose transport units from within an intracellular pool so that total glucose transport capacity is increased. Insulin also increases muscle glucose phosphorylation, glycogen synthesis and glycolysis by mechanisms similar to those found in liver.

Actions on lipid metabolism are less pronounced than in liver, but effects on protein metabolism are important. The uptake of amino acids is increased, particularly neutral amino acids, and insulin has a major stimulating effect on protein synthesis. It may also have a direct effect in inhibiting proteolysis.

Adipose tissue

In normal adipose tissue there is a balance between lipolysis, with hormone-sensitive lipase the key enzyme, and re-esterification. For this, new α-glycerophosphate must be synthesised via glycolysis. Since glucose entry into adipose tissue is insulin-dependent, insulin plays a major role in these processes. Glycolysis is then promoted, leading to greater availability of α-glycerophosphate. Insulin may also directly enhance esterification. In man, unlike other species, insulin does not directly stimulate fatty acid synthesis in adipose tissue. Insulin also exerts an anticatabolic effect by inhibiting lipolysis through inhibition of hormone sensitive lipase.

Mechanism of Action of Insulin

The first step in the action of insulin is the binding of the hormone to a specific cell surface receptor. Such receptors have now been found on many tissues including the key metabolic tissues fat, muscle and liver, but also kidney, brain, placenta, endothelial cells, fibroblasts, monocytes, lymphocytes, erythrocytes, platelets and even spermatozoa.

Insulin receptors of different tissues have similar if not identical properties. The consensus at present is that the receptor is a transmembrane glycoprotein comprising two subunits of 125 000 molecular weight each and two smaller subunits of 90 000 molecular weight (Fig. 8.14). The receptors are found in clusters and show the property of negative cooperativity implying interaction between neighbouring binding sites depending on whether the receptors are occupied or not (there could, alternatively, be low and high affinity receptors, perhaps with different subunit structure).

The behaviour and number of insulin receptors do not remain static, but are subject to regulatory processes. Thus when circulating insulin levels are high, as for example in obesity, the number of receptors falls. This so-called 'down-regulation' may protect the cell against chronic overstimulation, and could explain many of the syndromes characterised by insulin resistance. Conversely, in insulin deficiency (e.g. untreated insulin-dependent diabetes), the number of receptors increases — 'up-regulation'. Receptor affinity for insulin may also be subject to acute regulation; glucocorticoids and a high carbohydrate intake decrease affinity, whilst fasting and acromegaly increase affinity. This may underlie the immediate and dramatic improvement in glycaemia observed when obese diabetics are fasted.

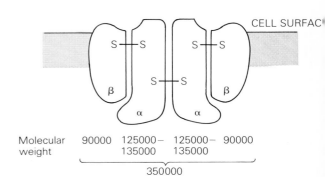

Fig. 8.14 *The structure of the insulin receptor.*

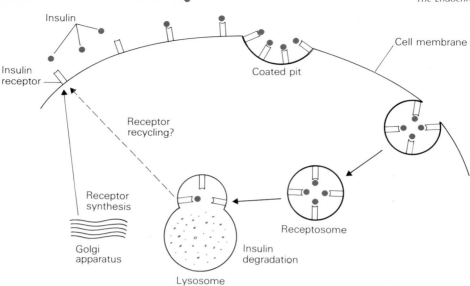

Fig. 8.15 *Internalization and recycling of the insulin receptor.*

Insulin receptors are not fixed components of the cell membrane but undergo a complex recycling process which can also explain the changes in receptor number which take place. Thus once the receptor binds an insulin molecule, the complex is internalised by the cell (Fig. 8.15) following clustering in special membrane pits. The pits form vesicles, receptosomes (or endosomes), which pass into the cell cytosol and Golgi apparatus. The insulin is detached and degraded, probably by lysosomes, and this forms the most important site of insulin degradation, whilst the receptors either recycle back to the membrane or are also degraded. Insulin reaches the liver via the portal vein in concentrations far in excess of peripheral levels because the liver actively binds about half of the insulin reaching it (the exact proportion depends on nutritional state and input), which is then internalised and degraded. This has important physiological connotations in terms of tissue metabolism of ingested nutrients.

Although much is now known about the insulin receptor there is considerable argument regarding the mechanism whereby combination of insulin with its receptor triggers the biological events within the cell — the actions described above. The initial hypothesis was that insulin activated adenyl cyclase and hence increased intracellular cyclic AMP concentration. More recently changes in intracellular calcium distribution have been implicated, as has a peptide mediator which may be released from the cell surface. The situation has been clarified to some extent by the discovery that insulin causes phosphorylation of its own receptor. The receptor itself is a protein kinase which is activated five- or six-fold by insulin binding. This has several important implications. First, it is in line with the actions of other hormones, such as adrenaline. Second, it obviates the need for a 'second messenger' for insulin action. There is still uncertainty however, about the nature of the substrate linking the receptor kinase and enzyme activation. In any case it is now clear that cyclic AMP and calmodulin protein kinases are not involved, and that the receptor kinase and perhaps a whole new family of kinases and phosphatases will turn out to be the missing links between the receptor and the final actions of insulin.

GLUCAGON

Glucagon forms one of the group of anti-insulin or catabolic hormones which together oppose the actions of insulin. Glucagon, originally discovered as a minor contaminant of early insulin preparations, has its primary actions on the liver.

Chemistry, Biosynthesis, Storage and Release

Glucagon has a molecular weight of 3485. It consists of one chain of 29 amino acids, quite different from that of insulin (Fig. 8.16). The gastrointestinal tract contains molecules which cross-react immunologically with glucagon. One appears to be immunologically identical and to have the same molecular size as pancreatic glucagon. It has been identified in cells of the stomach which cannot be distinguished from A cells of the pancreas. Glycentin is another gut molecule with glucagon-like immunoreactivity (GLI) which is found in cells in the small and large intestine and consists of glucagon with a C terminal extension of 1500 daltons.

It is believed that a similar synthetic sequence for glucagon occurs in the pancreatic A cell as for insulin in the B cell, and there is evidence for several large-molecular-weight precursors (proglucagons). Again, as for insulin, both calcium and cyclic AMP have been implicated in the regulation of glucagon secretion.

The measurement of glucagon in plasma has presented more difficulty than that of insulin, since antibodies to pancreatic glucagon often cross-react with gut glucagons. Moreover, plasma contains an enzyme degrading system which rapidly inactivates glucagon. Like insulin, 50% of the glucagon secreted into the portal vein is removed in a single passage through the liver, giving low concentrations in the peripheral blood. For these reasons progress has been slow in unravelling the physiology of glucagon secretion and there is still uncertainty about the absolute concentration of glucagon in plasma.

Factors Directly Affecting the Secretion of Glucagon

Substrates

The secretion of glucagon is suppressed by glucose. Conversely, a low blood concentration of glucose stimulates its release.

Amino acids provide the other main stimulus to glucagon secretion. Major differences in the ability of individual amino acids to stimulate glucagon release are unrelated to their ability to stimulate insulin secretion. Arginine is the most potent for both, but leucine, a good insulin stimulator, does not stimulate the secretion of glucagon, and alanine, the major gluconeogenic precursor, stimulates glucagon but not insulin.

Glucagon secretion is suppressed by high and stimulated by low concentration of fatty acids.

Pancreatic hormones

The secretion of glucagon is suppressed directly (independently of glucose) by insulin.

Gastrointestinal hormones

Cholecystokinin (CCK) is a potent stimulator of glucagon secretion. Since it is released during absorption of

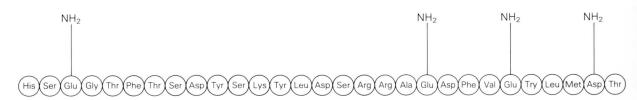

Fig. 8.16 *Structure of glucagon.*

protein, it is believed to have an important role in transmitting information from the gastrointestinal tract to the islets and in synchronising absorption and storage of amino acids. Other gut hormones, including gastrin and GIP, have similar effects.

α-Adrenoceptor agonists

Release of glucagon is stimulated by both adrenaline and noradrenaline at the physiological concentration seen in stress situations *in vivo*.

In contrast to the well-accepted alpha-adrenergic inhibition and beta stimulation of B and D cells, there is disagreement about A cell adrenoceptor mechanisms.

Cholinergic agents

Glucagon secretion is increased by acetylcholine and stimulation of the parasympathetic. Patients with truncal vagotomy have a reduced glucagon response to hypoglycaemia.

Actions of Glucagon

The major effects of glucagon are summarised in Table 8.4. These include acute stimulation of glycogenolysis and a more chronic effect in stimulating gluconeogenesis, through inhibition of pyruvate kinase, increasing flow of three carbon units from pyruvate through oxaloacetate and back to phosphoenolpyruvate, and presumed activation of fructose 1,6-diphosphatase and glucose 6-phosphatase. Some of these actions are mediated through stimulation of fructose 2,6-diphosphate production. At the same time glucagon specifically stimulates the uptake of alanine by the liver (one of the key gluconeogenic amino acids).

Glucagon also influences hepatic lipid metabolism. First there is inhibition of acetyl CoA carboxylase, slowing fatty acid synthesis and causing a fall of malonyl CoA concentration and hence activation of the carnitine shuttle (Fig. 8.17). Fatty acyl CoA molecules are therefore directed into mitochondria where they undergo β-oxidation to acetyl CoA and, ultimately, the ketone bodies, acetoacetate and 3-hydroxybutyrate, via the 3-hydroxy-3-methylglutaryl CoA pathway. Finally, glucagon may well increase lipolysis

Table 8.4

Main Actions of Glucagon

Carbohydrate metabolism	
Gluconeogenesis	+
Glycogenolysis (liver)	+
Lipid metabolism	
Ketogenesis	+
Liver lipoprotein release	−
*Lipolysis	+
Protein metabolism	
Protein synthesis (liver)	−
Amino acid transport (liver)	+
Ureagenesis	+

+ Indicates increase; − indicates decrease.
* Only effective in absence of insulin.

of intrahepatic triglycerides, and also inhibits secretion of VLDL.

When insulin is deficient, glucagon increases adipose tissue lipolysis by activating hormone-sensitive lipase thereby increasing the flow of fatty-acid substrate to the liver. This effect is, however, overcome by small amounts of insulin.

The suggestion that the 'glucagon:insulin ratio' is a key determinant of substrate flow within tissues should be viewed as an oversimplification, since it ignores the effects of the other anti-insulin hormones (see below).

Mechanism of Action of Glucagon

Like insulin, glucagon binds to a cell surface protein receptor which is also subject to 'up' and 'down' regulation depending on circulating hormone concentrations. In this case, however, the receptor is attached through a modulator GTP-binding protein to the adenyl cyclase complex. The net result is of glucagon binding to the receptor, activation of adenyl cyclase, release of cyclic AMP and activation of the cyclic AMP specific − protein kinase. This in turn causes phosphorylation and activation of a series of degradative enzymes. The classic example is the enzyme cascade resulting in glycogenolysis (Fig. 8.18).

HEPATOCYTE

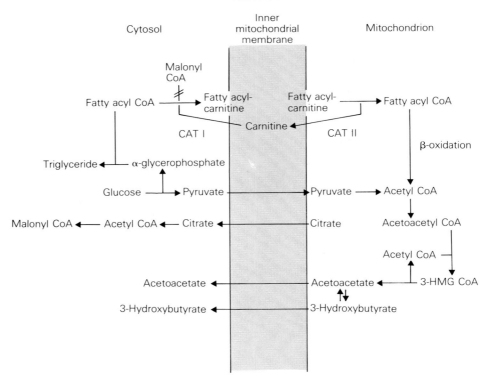

Fig. 8.17 *The carnitine shuttle.*

SOMATOSTATIN

Somatostatin, originally discovered as a hypothalamic growth hormone release inhibiting factor, has subsequently been found in many tissues, including the D cells of the islets of Langerhans.

Somatostatin Structure, Synthesis, Storage and Release

Somatostatin is a 14-amino-acid cyclic polypeptide with a 12-membered ring joined by disulphide bonds between 2 cysteine residues. It has a molecular weight of 1639 (Fig. 8.19). It is present in many neurones including those of the hypothalamus, midbrain, cortex,

pons, cerebellum and spinal cord, in the parafollicular cells of the thyroid, and in D-like cells in the gastrointestinal tract, as well as in the D cells of the pancreatic islets. Unlike A and PP cells, B and D cells are present in a constant ratio in all islets. Somatostatin biosynthesis and release is thought to be similar to that of insulin and a large precursor molecule has been demonstrated.

Unlike insulin and glucagon, somatostatin immunoreactivity exists in both bound and free forms in plasma, which complicates immunoassay. Moreover, plasma contains proteolytic enzymes which destroy somatostatin unless special precautions are taken in processing samples.. These methodological problems probably explain the discrepancies in values reported for the concentration of somatostatin in peripheral blood. Its half-life is about 1–2 minutes, and the liver, muscles and kidneys seem to be the major sites of degradation.

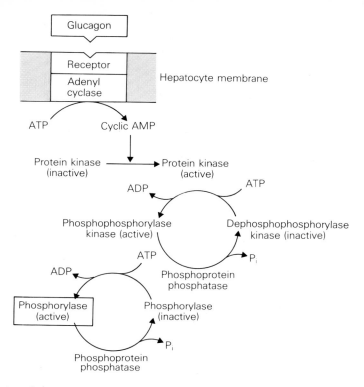

Fig. 8.18 *Mechanism of action of glucagon.*

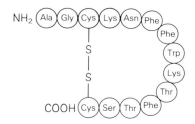

Fig. 8.19 *Structure of somatostatin.*

Factors Directly Affecting the Secretion of Somatostatin

Substrates

Glucose, arginine, leucine and ketoisocaproic acid stimulate the biphasic release of somatostatin, whereas D-glyceraldehyde inhibits it. The pancreatic D cell seems to be less sensitive to glucose than are the A and B cells.

Pancreatic hormones

Low concentrations of glucagon (< 1 ng/ml) stimulates the biphasic release of somatostatin. Insulin does not affect the secretion of somatostatin.

Gastrointestinal hormones

GIP, CCK, serotonin and VIP stimulate somatostatin secretion.

Neural control

Secretion of somatostatin is increased by beta-adrenergic stimulation and decreased by alpha-adrenergic stimulation, acetylcholine and dopamine.

Actions of Somatostatin

Somatostatin is probably important as a paracrine substance with an additional role as a neurotransmitter rather than as a circulating hormone. It is a potent inhibitor of secretion of several hormones, including the pancreatic hormones insulin and glucagon and the pituitary hormones, growth hormone and TSH. It also decreases splanchnic blood-flow and gastric-acid secretion. The physiological role of somatostatin is not clearly established, and its mechanism of action remains elusive.

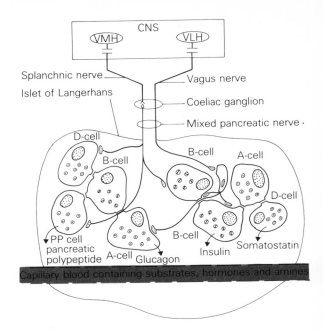

Fig. 8.20 *Central connections and pathways for the autonomic regulation of the endocrine pancreas.*

PANCREATIC POLYPEPTIDE

Structure, Synthesis, Storage and Release

Although present almost exclusively in the PP cells of the pancreas, this 36-amino-acid polypeptide (molecular weight 4200) seems to function largely as a gastrointestinal hormone.

Little is known about its synthesis, storage and degradation, but a marked increase lasting for several hours occurs in plasma PP after ingestion of protein, and this response is mediated by the vagus. A smaller and shorter rise occurs following ingestion of glucose and triglyceride. Its action is unknown.

THE ISLET AS AN INTEGRATOR

The secretion of insulin, glucagon and somatostatin is under the control of all three dietary nutrients, glucose, free fatty acids and amino acids, with glucose playing a key permissive role. Transplanted isolated islets function well and can maintain a normal, or near normal, metabolism, indicating that neural activity is not essential and that fluctuation of the level of nutrients during and after meals accounts for most instances of altered hormone secretion.

However, in the intact animal two systems of modulation exist which allow it to refine and tune its metabolic adaptation to the environment. Thus, extra-pancreatic hormones such as thyroid hormones, gluco-corticoids, oestrogens, progesterone, somatomedins and gut hormones (GIP, CCK, secretin and gastrin) alter islet function by signalling general metabolic needs, while needs perceived by the CNS are communicated directly by nerves and by neuro- and other transmitters within the islets. This neuroendocrine modulation provides the background from which the islet cells respond to nutrients (Fig. 8.20).

INTEGRATED REGULATION OF METABOLISM

Basal State

Regulation of metabolism in the basal state maintains a continuous supply of suitable substrate to body cells (Fig. 8.21). Certain tissues, e.g. nerves, red cells and renal medulla, have an obligatory requirement for glucose; other tissues can metabolise a wide variety of substrates such as non-esterified fatty acids, ketone bodies and lactate. In chronic fasting, some parts of the nervous system are able to utilise ketone bodies.

Between 180–260 g/24 hrs glucose is used in the basal state, of which between one-half and one-third is accounted for by the brain. Initially hepatic glycogen provides the bulk of this but stores are limited (approx. 60 g after an overnight fast) and rapidly depleted. Muscle glycogen can also add indirectly to the glucose pool by glycolysis to pyruvate, the release of lactate and pyruvate into the circulation and their re-incorporation into glucose. Muscle lactate, plus lactate from other tissues, forms approximately 50% of the gluconeogenic precursors used by the liver. In the basal state, only the liver contributes significantly to the

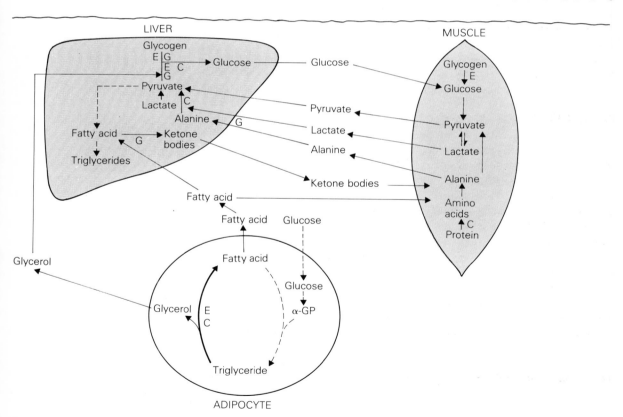

Fig. 8.21 *Integrated regulation of metabolism in the basal (fasting) state. E = adrenaline; C = cortisol; G = glucagon.*

Table 8.5

*Levels of Circulating Substrates in Different
Nutritional States in Man*

| | Fed | Starvation | | |
		12 hrs	24 hrs	48 hrs
Glucose mM	5.5–8	4.0–5.5	3.5–5.0	3.0–5.0
Lactate mM	0.8–1.5	0.4–0.9	0.4–0.8	0.4–0.8
Alanine mM	0.30–0.40	0.25–0.35	0.2–0.3	0.15–0.2
Glycerol mM	0.02–0.04	0.04–0.07	0.05–0.1	0.08–0.14
Non-esterified fatty acids mM	0.1–0.4	0.3–0.8	0.6–1.0	0.8–1.3
Total ketone bodies mM	0.01–0.02	0.02–0.2	0.1–0.5	0.4–1.2

glucose pool, with the kidney producing approximately 10%. This is because tissues other than liver and kidney lack the key enzyme glucose 6-phosphatase. As starvation progresses, the kidney may be responsible for up to 50% of gluconeogenesis.

Gluconeogenesis must use substrates other than lactate: from adipose tissue lipolysis, glycerol provides 10% whilst the remaining 40% comes from amino acids. Proteolysis occurs in peripheral tissues, where alanine and glutamine are the predominant amino acids released. Obviously carbon skeletons of amino acids must also be delivered from the periphery or else no net gluconeogenesis would occur from amino acids. As fasting progresses so the need for glucose decreases due to increased utilisation of lipid substrates. This results in diminished need for amino acids so that body protein is preserved. Ketone bodies seem to inhibit proteolysis, thus aiding in protein preservation.

In the basal state adipose tissue lipolysis increases, resulting in increased release of non-esterified fatty acids into the circulation. These serve as fuels in many tissues, but are also extracted by the liver and converted into ketone bodies which (since they cannot be used directly by the liver due to lack of the appropriate enzyme) pass into the circulation for use in tissues such as heart, muscle, gut and — if starvation is prolonged — brain. Table 8.5 shows circulating levels of different substrates and precursors at different stages of the fed and fasting state. This emphasises the relative constancy of blood glucose levels whilst lipid substrates show marked fluctuations depending on the nutritional state.

All these processes are under fine control by hormones. Insulin secretion is low in the basal state but levels are adequate to exert the anticatabolic effects of the hormone; i.e. a restraining partial inhibitory effect on glycogenolysis, gluconeogenesis, lipolysis and proteolysis. Thus none of these catabolic processes run amok. At the same time there is a relative excess of cortisol, promoting proteolysis, hepatic conversion of amino acids into glucose precursor intermediates, and gluconeogenesis, of glucagon promoting glycogenolysis and gluconeogenesis, and of catecholamines increasing adipose tissue lipolysis, muscle and liver glycogenolysis and hepatic gluconeogenesis. Cortisol and adrenaline also inhibit glucose uptake by muscle and adipose tissue, whilst insulin levels are too low to promote glucose uptake, so that glucose supplies are preserved. Glucagon, together with low insulin levels, also promotes the activation of muscle endothelial lipoprotein lipase so that more fatty acid substrate is delivered to muscle as a food source.

The Fed State

In the fed state, there is a need for rapid anabolism so that fuels can be stored for later use. After an average mixed meal approximately 60% of ingested carbohydrate is taken up by the liver, either in the form of glucose, or as fructose (from sucrose) and galactose (from lactose) which are then converted to glucose. Some glucose is converted to glycogen, and the rest is converted to fatty acids, esterified to triglycerides and exported as VLDL. The remaining 40% of glucose is used as oxidisable fuel by extrahepatic tissues and also serves to replenish extrahepatic glycogen stores.

Ingested amino acids serve to replenish tissue amino acid stores, and excess amino acids (except branched-chain amino acids) are extracted by the liver, de-aminated and the carbon skeletons used for lipid synthesis.

Fats are absorbed from the gut as fatty acids or monoglycerides. Short-chain fatty acids pass directly to the liver via the portal venous system whilst the longer-chain fatty acids are reformed into triglycerides and subsequently incorporated into chylomicrons in the intestinal mucosa. They then pass via the lymphatic system into the systemic circulation. In the fed state, adipose tissue endothelial lipoprotein lipase is activated and fatty acids are removed both from chylomicrons and VLDL and diffuse into adipose tissue where they are esterified and laid down as triglyceride stores.

Again the hormonal milieu is all important in determining the direction of substrate flow in the fed state. Insulin, the prime anabolic hormone, will be present in a relative excess compared with the cata-bolic hormones. After meals peripheral levels of 30–80 μU/ml are found (basal values 4–10 μU/ml), with portal venous levels 2- to 5-fold higher. Secretion is stimulated by both glucose and amino acids. This explains the movement of glucose into muscle and adipose tissue, the stimulation of fatty acid synthesis, the laying down of triglyceride stores and the increase in protein synthesis. After a protein-containing meal, glucagon levels will also rise initially, thus preventing insulin-induced hypoglycaemia and allowing amino acids to be used for protein synthesis. When glucose levels rise, both glucagon and growth hormone secretion are rapidly inhibited. However, two to three hours after a meal, growth hormone levels rise, further promoting protein synthesis. Cortisol and adrenaline levels change little whilst the concentration of noradrenaline shows a small rise, the physiological significance of which remains unclear. The flow of substrates is much as that shown for the actions of insulin (Fig. 8.13). Figure 8.22 shows the hormonal response to a mixed meal and Table 8.5 the level of substrates in different nutritional states.

Exercise

Exercise represents a special stress, with a rapid increase in fuel demands. At rest, 90% of the energy requirements of muscle come from fatty acids and ketone bodies. In the initial stages of strenuous exercise,

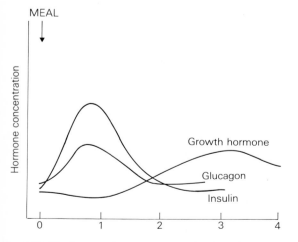

Fig. 8.22 *The hormonal response to a mixed meal.*

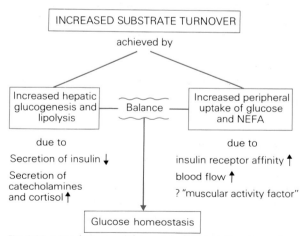

Fig. 8.23 *Main features of the metabolic adaptation to moderate exercise.*

energy comes from oxidation of stored glycogen but, if oxygen demands outstrip supply, anaerobic glycolysis becomes all-important. Glycogen supplies are rapidly depleted, and glucose is extracted from the circulation independent of insulin. Blood glucose levels tend to fall and insulin secretion also decreases. Catecholamine and cortisol levels rise, stimulating lipolysis and gluconeogenesis. The increase in hepatic glucose production matches the increased extrahepatic utilisation so that glucose levels do not change markedly (Fig. 8.23). As anaerobic glycolysis continues, so blood lactate levels rise, reaching 10–12 mmol/l in strenuous exercise (normal basal values, 0.4–1.0 mmol/l). This lactate is recycled by the liver as new glucose. When exercise stops there is a small rebound in glucose and ketone body levels; lactate levels fall gradually back to normal, whilst both anabolic and catabolic hormone secretion is also rapidly restored to normal levels.

The Metabolic Effects of Insulin Deficiency

The effects of insulin deficiency may be predicted from the actions of insulin described above (Fig. 8.13, Table 8.3). Insulin exerts its anticatabolic effects at a lower concentration than that required for its anabolic actions. This means that when insulin deficiency is partial, as in patients with non-insulin-dependent

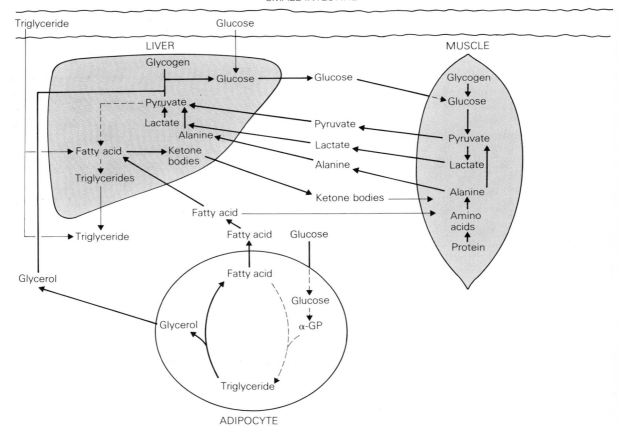

Fig. 8.24 *The metabolic effects of insulin deficiency. Dotted lines indicate inhibited pathways.*

diabetes, the anticatabolic effect of insulin may be relatively well preserved while its anabolic action is more seriously defective. In these circumstances lipolysis is not markedly accelerated, the concentration of ketone bodies in the blood remains normal or near normal, the fasting blood glucose concentration and hepatic gluconeogenesis are only moderately increased, and body protein is largely preserved. The disposal of ingested food is, however, seriously impaired so that there is a marked rise in the post-prandial blood concentration of glucose, triglyceride (due to defective clearance of circulating chylomicrons by adipose tissue lipoprotein lipase) and amino acids.

In total insulin deficiency a much more serious metabolic derangement occurs which, without treatment, leads inexorably to death from diabetic ketoacidosis (Fig. 8.24). Loss of the anticatabolic effects of insulin results in unrestrained glycogenolysis and greatly accelerated gluconeogenesis and lipolysis.

Glucose is no longer taken up by insulin-dependent tissues so that progressively more glucose accumulates in the extracellular fluid (ECF). This leads to: 1. ECF hyperosmolality with loss of intracellular fluid; 2. hyponatraemia as glucose replaces sodium as ECF 'osmoles'; 3. osmotic diuresis with loss of water and electrolytes (sodium, potassium, chloride, phosphate, magnesium and calcium), with signs of obvious dehydration; and 4. hypovolaemia with hypotension and tachycardia.

Similarly, adipose tissue lipolysis is accelerated and re-esterification inhibited so that progressively more fatty acids (and glycerol) are released from adipose tissue. The fatty acids are taken up by the liver and, again because of insulin lack and the unopposed actions of glucagon, enter into mitochondria, undergo β-oxidation and form ketone bodies which are released into the circulation. Production far exceeds utilisation so that levels of blood ketone bodies may rise as much as 200-fold. The ketone bodies (which are acids) dissociate almost completely at physiological pH, producing a marked excess of H^+ ions. Initially the body responds with marked hyperventilation and bicarbonate levels fall. Soon, however, buffering and excretory capacities are exceeded and extracellular pH falls. Hydrogen ions move into cells, with potassium moving out in exchange and ultimately being lost in urine. The acidaemia also has negative inotropic effects on the heart and causes peripheral vasodilation, further worsening hypotension and causing hypothermia. Vomiting also occurs, further worsening the fluid and electrolyte deficits.

Insulin deficiency alone may cause these changes. The situation is, however, further exacerbated by the increased secretion of HGH, glucagon, cortisol and ultimately catecholamines which inevitably follows insulin deficiency. Partial insulin deficiency can be converted into an effectively total deficiency by any illness, e.g. an infection which causes increased secretion of the catabolic hormones.

EFFECT OF INSULIN EXCESS

The Metabolic Effects of Insulin Excess

Since glucose is the only metabolic fuel used by the central nervous system under most conditions encountered in normal life, and the brain can neither synthesise nor store glucose, an array of mechanisms exists in the normal animal to ensure that the arterial blood glucose concentration is maintained above 2.5 mmol/l. In normal subjects, administration of exogenous insulin causes hypoglycaemia which is followed by a rapid increase in the secretion of glucagon, growth hormone, cortisol and catecholamines (Fig. 8.25). Glucagon normally plays the primary role in raising the blood glucose concentration but deficiency of glucagon can be largely compensated for by increased secretion of adrenaline. Only in the absence of both these hormones does glucose recovery fail to occur. Neither growth hormone nor cortisol appear to be critical in the recovery from acute insulin-induced hypoglycaemia although chronic deficiency may lead to fasting hypoglycaemia. The probable actions of the hormones countering the effects of insulin ('counter-regulatory hormones') are shown in Table 8.6.

DIABETES MELLITUS

Diabetes mellitus is a clinical syndrome characterised by hyperglycaemia. This can arise in many different ways and the diagnostic label thus embraces numerous different disorders (Table 8.7).

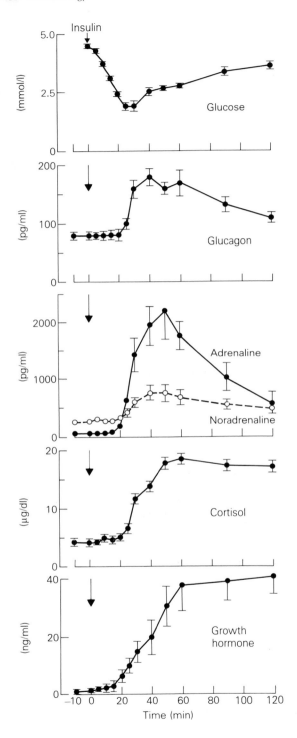

Epidemiological studies of whole populations have shown that the distribution of blood glucose concentration, i.e. carbohydrate tolerance, is unimodal, with no clear division between normal and abnormal values. Diagnostic criteria are therefore arbitrary. Population studies involving the Pima Indians in Arizona and the civil servants in Whitehall have shown that hyperglycaemia represents an independent risk factor for the development of disease of small and large blood vessels respectively. Current diagnostic criteria for diabetes (Table 8.8) have been selected on the basis of identifying those who have a degree of hyperglycaemia which has been shown to be associated with an increased risk of disability and death from vascular disease, irrespective of the basic cause of the hyperglycaemia.

Classification of Diabetes

Two main categories of diabetes are recognised: primary (idiopathic) and secondary diabetes. The majority of cases seen belong to the former group, which in turn consists of two main clinical types: insulin-dependent diabetes mellitus (IDDM), i.e. those who, without the administration of exogenous insulin, die rapidly in ketoacidosis, and non-insulin-dependent diabetes mellitus (NIDDM), i.e. those who can survive without treatment with insulin. There is a close correlation between the clinical type of diabetes, the treatment required, the concentration of insulin in plasma, and the pathological changes seen in the pancreatic islets. IDDM is characterised by an absolute and NIDDM by a relative deficiency of endogenous insulin (Fig. 8.26). IDDM is associated with the virtual disappearance of B cells from the islets, combined with evidence of excessive activity (nuclear enlargement and cytoplasmic degranulation) in the few B cells which remain. In contrast, in NIDDM the relative and absolute volume of all cell types appears to be within the normal range.

Until recently, the spectrum of insulin deficiency seen in clinical diabetes was assumed to represent

Fig. 8.25 *Changes in the mean (±SEM) plasma concentration of glucose and counterregulatory hormones in normal men.*

Table 8.6

Probable Actions of Hormones Countering the Effect of Insulin in Man

	Insulin release	Muscle glucose uptake	Hepatic glucogenesis	Ketogenesis	Lipolysis	Proteolysis
Catecholamines	↓	↓	↑	↑	↑	↑
Glucagon	–	–	↑	↑	–	–
Growth hormone	–	↓	–	↑	↑	↓
Glucocorticoids	–	–	↑	↑	↑	↑
Thyroid hormones	–	–	↑	↑	↑	↑

↑ = increase; ↓ = decrease; – = no significant primary effect.

Table 8.7

Classification of Diabetes Mellitus

A   *Primary (Idiopathic)*
   Type 1   Insulin-dependent diabetes mellitus (IDDM)
   Type 2   Non-insulin-dependent diabetes mellitus (NIDDM)

B   *Secondary to other pathology*   *Examples*
   1. Pancreatic pathology   pancreatitis
                                             haemochromatosis
                                             neoplastic disease
                                             pancreatectomy
                                             cystic fibrosis

   *2. Excess endogenous production
   of hormonal antagonists to
   insulin*   growth hormone (acromegaly)
                                             glucocorticoids (Cushing's syndrome)
                                             thyroid hormones (hyperthyroidism)
                                             catecholamines (phaeochromocytoma)
                                             HPL (pregnancy)
                                             glucagon (glucagonoma)
                                             severe burns (glucagon, cortisol,
                                                 catecholamines)
   3. Medication with   corticosteroids
                                             thiazide diurectics
                                             phenytoin

   4. Liver disease

C   *Associated with genetic syndromes*   DIDMOAD (i.e. diabetes insipidus, diabetes
                                                 mellitus, optic atrophy, nerve deafness)
                                             lipoatrophy
                                             muscular dystrophies
                                             Friedreich's ataxia
                                             Down's syndrome
                                             Klinefelter's syndrome
                                             Turner's syndrome

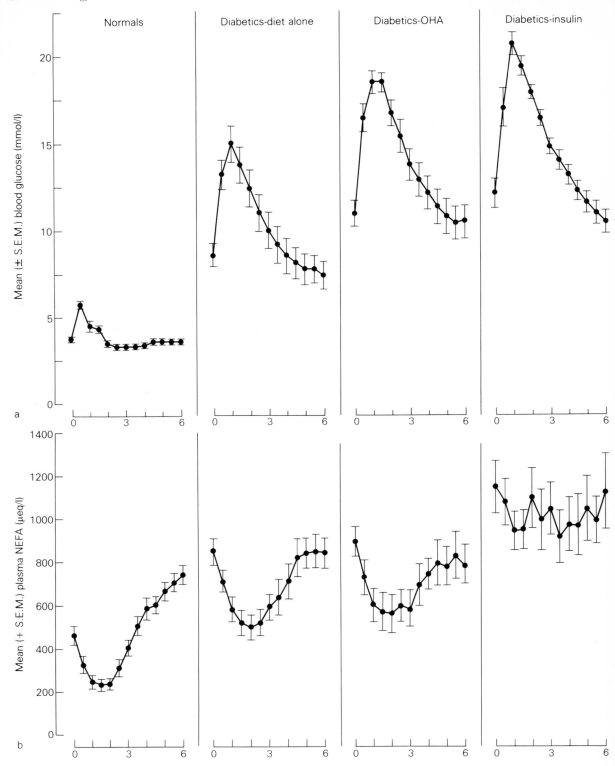

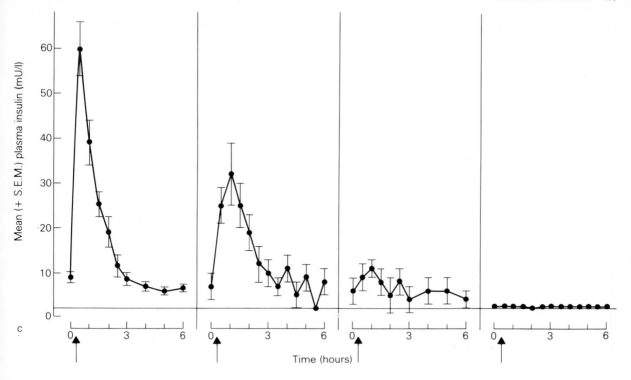

Fig. 8.26 Mean (±SEM) plasma concentration of glucose, non-esterified fatty acids, and immunoreactive insulin in the fasting state and at half-hourly intervals after 50 g glucose orally (indicated by ↑) in normal subjects and in newly diagnosed untreated diabetic patients grouped on the basis of the treatment they were subsequently found to require on clinical grounds. The solid line at the foot of the section relating to insulin secretion indicates the lower limit of sensitivity of the assay.

Table 8.8

Diagnostic Criteria for Diabetes Mellitus (WHO 1985)

| | Glucose concentration mmol/l (mg/100 ml) | |
	Normal	Diabetic
Fasting	< 5.6 (100)	> 6.7 (120)
2 hours after 75 g glucose orally	< 6.7 (120)	> 10.0 (180)

Note—These figures refer to the concentration of glucose in venous whole blood (estimated by a specific enzymatic assay). Values for plasma glucose are about 15% higher than those for whole blood. Intermediate readings indicate the need for further evaluation of the patient including the history obtained. In pregnancy those with intermediate readings should be treated as diabetic.

degrees of severity of a single disorder. Advances in understanding have stemmed from appreciation of the fundamental point that in all types of diabetes it is the tendency to develop diabetes, rather than diabetes *per se*, which is inherited and that the action of additional environmental factors is required for clinical expression of the genetic susceptibility. It is clear that IDDM and NIDDM are aetiologically distinct and separate disorders with different patterns of inheritance and precipitating environmental factors.

Aetiology of IDDM

In 1974 it was found that the frequency of certain histocompatibility antigens (B8 and B15) was increased in patients with IDDM. Since then there has been an explosion of work in this field. The current position is summarised in Fig. 8.27.

The increased risk of developing IDDM is primarily associated with the D locus, and associations with alleles at the A, C, B, Bf, C2 and the two C4 loci occur because of linkage disequilibrium (i.e. the tendency for alleles at different loci to occur together more often in the same haplotype than is expected by chance). There are two established axes of susceptibility: one associated with DW3, DR3 and one with DW4, DR4. The

Table 8.9

Relative Risk of Developing IDDM Conferred by HLA–DR Antigens

HLA–DR	Relative risk	95% confidence limits
DR2	0.12	0.05–0.31
DR3	7.39	4.13–13.22
DR4	9.25	5.03–17.02
DR7	0.12	0.05–0.27
DR3, DR4	14.26	6.25–32.41
DR3, DR	0.80	0.43–1.48
DR4, DR	0.95	0.53–1.68
DR, DR	0.04	0.01–0.13

Note—DR includes DR1, DR2, DR5, DRW6, DR7, DRW8, DRW9, and DRW10.
(Data of Cudworth and Wolf, 1982)

frequencies and relative risks for the relevant antigens associated with diabetes are shown in Table 8.9.

The HLA DR determinants are probably in turn in linkage disequilibrium with immune respone (Ir) genes which, it is postulated, exist on chromosome 6 within the HLA region. Since there is at present no way of defining Ir genes in man, the HLA antigens serve as 'markers' for them. The existence of Ir genes has been validated in the mouse, where there are several well-defined Ir regions within the H2 complex — the major histocompatibility system in this animal.

Various hypotheses have been proposed to explain

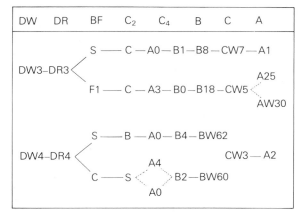

Fig. 8.27 *The two established axes of susceptibility for IDDM within the HLA complex.*

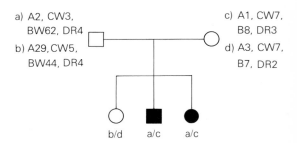

a) A2, CW3, BW62, DR4
b) A29, CW5, BW44, DR4
c) A1, CW7, B8, DR3
d) A3, CW7, B7, DR2

Fig. 8.28 *HLA genotypes in a family with two insulin-dependent diabetic children. The paternal haplotypes are indicated as a, b and the maternal as c, d. The two affected children are HLA identical whereas the unaffected child has inherited the alternative parental haplotypes.*

Table 8.10

Heterogeneity Within Type I Diabetes

	Type IA	Type IB
HLA link	DW4, DR4	DW3, DR3
Linkage disequilibrium	A2, B15, B40, CW3	A1, B8, B18
Aetiology	Viral	Autoimmune
	? role of food additives and contaminants	
Islet cell antibody	Transient	Persistent
Antipancreatic cell-mediated immunity	No	Yes
Tendency to develop antibodies to exogenous insulin	Increased	Decreased
Susceptibility to develop diabetic complications	Not increased	Increased
Associated with other autoimmune disease*	No	Yes
Age	Younger	Any age
Sex preponderance	Male	Female

* e.g. thyroid disease (both hyper- and hypothyroidism), Addison's disease, pernicious anaemia.

linkage disequilibrium. The most likely explanation is that natural selection has favoured the persistence of groups of HLA genes which may have afforded protection against environmental factors or disease that threatened survival of a species in the past. Subjects who are DW2, DR2 with secondary associations with A3 and B7 have a significantly reduced risk of developing IDDM, possibly because of linkage disequilibrium with genes which confer resistance. Affected siblings of diabetics also usually have one, and in many cases both, haplotypes in common, irrespective of the HLA determinants that make up the haplotype (Fig. 8.28).

The mode of action of these genes remains speculative. It is is probable that they control the immune response to environmental factors capable of initiating damage to the pancreatic islet B cell membrane. It is postulated that susceptible individuals react abnormally to assaults by viruses or cytotoxic agents, and the presence of islet cell antibodies in the plasma of 80% of newly-diagnosed IDD patients suggests that autoimmune phenomena may be involved in the mechanism of loss of pancreatic B cells. Prospective family studies suggest that an immune-mediated destruction of the B cell involving both humoral and cell-mediated immunological processes occurs slowly over several years prior to the development of clinical diabetes. This long pre-diabetic period suggests the possibility of preventing the development of clinical IDDM by arresting the destructive process through manipulation of the immune system before 90% of the pancreatic B cell mass has been obliterated. Indeed amelioration of diabetes has recently been demonstrated in preliminary studies in which cyclosporin was given to newly-diagnosed insulin-dependent diabetic patients.

There seems little doubt that there is a slight, but definite, male excess (12–20%) in IDDM developing in young people. It is interesting that male children are also known to be more susceptible to certain viruses such as polio and some coxsackie B4 viruses.

The concept of two separate HLA DR associated susceptibility genes suggests the possibility of separate associations between DR3 and DR4 and immunological or clinical aspects of the disease. Table 8.10 provides some evidence of heterogeneity within IDDM.

Aetiology of NIDDM

NIDDM is not HLA-linked and there is no evidence that autoimmunity or viruses have anything to do with its development. Studies with twins and sibships show that genetic factors are more important in the development of NIDDM than in IDDM but there is little information about what is inherited.

Recently the insulin gene, situated on the short arm of chromosome 11 in man, has been investigated as a possible genetic marker for NIDDM. Using restriction enzymes, three alleles of the insulin gene have been demonstrated: an upper allele (UU), a lower allele (LL) and a third allele which is a mixture of the other two sequences (UL). A significant increase has been demonstrated in the frequency of the UU allele in NIDDM compared with IDDM patients, and non-diabetic carriers of the UU allele show a delayed insulin response to oral glucose and reduced glucose tolerance with age. However, although the UU allele seems to affect blood glucose homeostasis its relationship to the development of NIDDM is uncertain.

Simple deficiency of insulin cannot entirely account for the diabetic syndrome in NIDDM. Increased hepatic production of glucose and resistance to the action of insulin are characteristic features of this disorder. Insulin resistance is also seen in obesity which so often accompanies NIDDM. However, many non-obese, non-insulin-dependent patients are also insulin resistant. Insulin resistance may be due to any of three general causes (Table 8.11).

Target tissue defects are the common cause of insulin resistance in NIDDM. The specific mechanisms underlying this insulin resistant state are heterogeneous. In patients with relatively mild impairment of carbohydrate tolerance the defect in insulin action may be due mainly to a decreased number of cellular insulin receptors. Patients with more severe hyperglycaemia usually combine a reduced number of receptors with a post-receptor defect in the action of insulin, and this seems to be the predominant abnormality. The relative role of receptor and post-receptor defects varies from case to case but, in general, as insulin resistance and hyperglycaemia increase, the post-receptor defect becomes more prominent.

Other types of insulin resistance are extremely rare.

Increased amounts of circulating hormonal antagonists are not thought to be primarily involved in the aetiology of either IDDM or NIDDM. However, uncontrolled diabetes, particularly IDDM, is associated with increased plasma levels of antistorage hormones, such as growth hormone and glucagon, and the normal suppressive effect of oral glucose on secretion of these hormones is diminished (p. 156). Treatment of the diabetes abolishes these abnormalities. Pregnancy is diabetogenic due to an increase in insulin antagonists, particularly human placental lactogen. A defective B cell may be unable to meet this demand and 'gestational diabetes' results.

Ketone bodies and non-esterified acids (NEFA) inhibit glucose utilisation by skeletal muscle *in vitro* and impair its sensitivity to insulin. In normal man, any situation leading to an increased rate of fatty acid oxidation tends to be associated with a decreased rate of glucose uptake and since most diabetic patients have an increased turnover of NEFA (Fig. 8.26), this is a potentially important mechanism contributing to their impaired carbohydrate tolerance.

It must be emphasised that increased hepatic production of glucose and/or decreased peripheral utilisation of glucose, alone or together, cannot lead to sustained hyperglycaemia unless the pancreatic islets fail to adapt to the situation. Inadequate adaptation of the islet in NIDDM may be due to B cell inhibitors, such as somatostatin, prostaglandin and serotonin, or other B cell secretory mechanisms may be impaired in these

---

Table 8.11

Possible Causes of Insulin Resistance

Abnormal B cell secretory product
   i. abnormal insulin molecule
   ii. incomplete conversion of proinsulin to insulin

Circulating insulin antagonists
   i. increased secretion of anti-storage hormones,
       e.g. GH, cortisol, glucagon, catecholamines
   ii. increased amounts of non-hormonal insulin antagonists,
       e.g. ketone bodies, NEFA
   iii. insulin antibodies
   iv. antibodies to insulin receptor

Target tissue defects
   i. insulin receptor defects
   ii. post-receptor defects

patients. Not only is the maximum absolute plasma insulin concentration reduced in most patients with NIDDM during an oral glucose tolerance test (Fig. 8.26), there is also a delay in the insulin response to glucose which is most clearly demonstrated when glucose is given intravenously (Fig. 8.11b). This indicates that the primary defect is in first phase secretion of insulin. However, both relative and absolute responses of insulin may be normal when challenged with arginine, secretin, isoprenaline (a β-adrenergic agonist) and tolbutamide. Therefore the defective insulin response appears to be selective for glucose. It is not known whether this B cell abnormality is due to intrinsic structural or metabolic change within the islet, or whether it is caused by some imbalance in neuroendocrine input or by a change in the sensitivity of the B cell to these stimuli, but some evidence exists in support of the latter concept.

EPIDEMIOLOGY

Diabetes is by far the most common of the endocrine disorders. It is worldwide in distribution and Table 8.12 shows that the prevalence of both IDDM and NIDDM varies considerably in different parts of the world. This seems to be due to differences in both genetic and environmental factors. The prevalence in Britain is between 1–2%, but almost half of NIDDM cases remain undetected.

The incidence of diabetes appears to be rising throughout the world. This can be partly attributed to the improved life expectancy of diabetic patients associated with better methods of treatment and higher standards of care, as well as to more diligent diagnosis. However, there is probably also a real rise in the incidence of diabetes, largely due to an increase in NIDDM.

Table 8.12

*Incidence and Prevalence of Diabetes
in Different Countries*

Insulin-dependent diabetes	Incidence per 100 000	Period of study	Prevalence per 100
Scotland	14	1968–1976	—
Northern England	10	1977–1979	—
Southern England	8	1977–1979	—
Netherlands	11	1978–1980	—
Norway	18	1973–1977	—
Finland	29	1970–1979	—
North Sweden	38	1973–1977	—
Rhode Island, USA	14	1979–1980	—
Kuwait	4	1980–1981	—
Denmark	— (all ages)	1973	0.33
England	— (0–26)	1946–1972	0.15
Non-insulin-dependent diabetes			
Northern England	17 (age 18–50)	1977–1979	—
Southern England	15 (age 18–50)	1977–1979	—
Nauru	1540	1980–1981	30.3
New Caledonia (Polynesia)			7.0
(Melanesian)			2.2
Malta		1978–1980	6.5
USA		1976–1980	6.7
Wadena, USA	101	1981	—

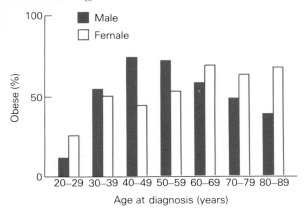

Fig. 8.29 *Distribution of all new cases of diabetes occurring within a defined geographical area over two years by age and obesity. Diabetic patients were classified as obese if they weighed 10% or more above the mean weight of all persons in the population of the same sex, height and age, or had been more than 10% overweight for more than half their adult life. This definition was employed to avoid underestimating the amount of obesity amongst these patients who often lose a large amount of weight as the disease is developing prior to the diagnosis being made.*

Risk Factors for NIDDM

Life style

Studies of the incidence of NIDDM provide evidence that overeating, especially when combined with obesity and underactivity, is related to the development of NIDDM. Middle-aged diabetic patients eat significantly more and are fatter and less active than their non-diabetic siblings. The majority of middle-aged diabetic patients are obese (Fig. 8.29) but only a few obese people develop diabetes. Obesity probably acts as a diabetogenic factor (through increasing resistance to the action of insulin, Fig. 8.30) in those genetically predisposed to develop NIDDM.

Age

In Britain over 70% of all cases of diabetes occur after the age of 50 years (Fig. 8.31). In contrast to IDDM which mainly affects younger people, NIDDM is principally a disease of the middle-aged and elderly (Fig. 8.32). Thus

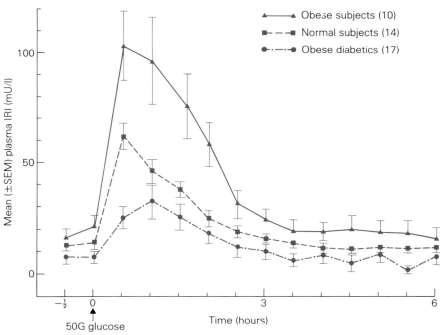

Fig. 8.30 *Mean (±SEM) plasma immunoreactive insulin concentration following ingestion of 50 g glucose by normal, thin adults, obese non-diabetics, and newly diagnosed, untreated, obese diabetic patients.*

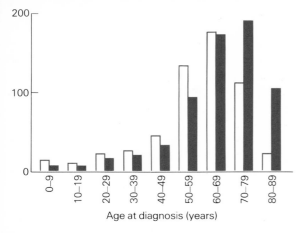

Fig. 8.31 *Age distribution of all new cases of diabetes mellitus occurring within a defined geographical area over two years. The clear columns represent the actual number of cases occurring in each 10 year age group; the black columns are the number of cases related to the total number of persons in the population at each age group, that is the relative annual incidence rate.*

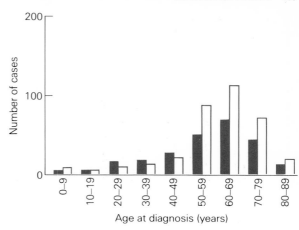

Fig. 8.33 *Distribution of all new cases of diabetes mellitus occurring within a defined geographical area over two years by age and sex. The clear columns represent the number of female cases.*

ageing is probably the most important risk factor of all for NIDDM.

Sex and pregnancy

There are rather more young male diabetics than female, but in middle age more females are affected (Fig. 8.33). During normal pregnancy the level of plasma insulin is raised by the action of placental hormones, thus placing a burden on the B cells of the pancreatic islets. A failing pancreas may be unable to meet these demands. The term 'gestational diabetes' refers to

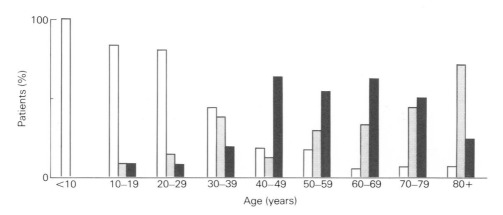

Fig. 8.32 *Treatment (at 3 months following diagnosis) and age of onset of diabetes in consecutive referrals to the Diabetic Clinic at the Western General Hospital, Edinburgh over a two year period. Patients with IDDM represented by clear bars, NIDDM patients taking an oral hypoglycaemic drug by hatched bars, and NIDDM patients treated by diet alone by solid bars.*

hyperglycaemia which may occur temporarily during pregnancy in the genetically predisposed. Repeated pregnancy may increase the likelihood of developing permanent diabetes, particularly in obese women.

Pathophysiology, Symptoms and Presentation

Whatever the aetiology, in all cases the hyperglycaemia of diabetes develops because of a relative or absolute deficiency of insulin which leads to 1. a reduced rate of removal of glucose from the blood by peripheral tissues, and 2. an increased rate of release of glucose from the liver into the circulation. When the concentration of glucose in the plasma exceeds the renal threshold (i.e. the capacity of renal tubules to reabsorb glucose from the glomerular filtrate), glyco-

suria occurs. The renal threshold is approximately 10 mmol/l, but there is wide individual variation.

Figure 8.34 relates the pathophysiology of diabetes to its symptoms. Note that the severity of the classical symptoms of diabetes, i.e. polyuria and polydipsia, is related directly to the degree of glycosuria. If hyperglycaemia develops slowly over many months or even years, as in NIDDM, the renal threshold for glucose rises; both glycosuria and the symptoms of diabetes are then correspondingly slight, which is one reason for the large number of undetected cases of NIDDM. Such individuals may have significant but symptomless hyperglycaemia for many years before glycosuria is noted on routine urine testing. Sometimes they eventually present with symptoms due to one or more of the complications of long-term diabetes — paraesthesiae, pain and muscle atrophy in the legs, or impotence due to neuropathy, deterioration of vision due to retino-

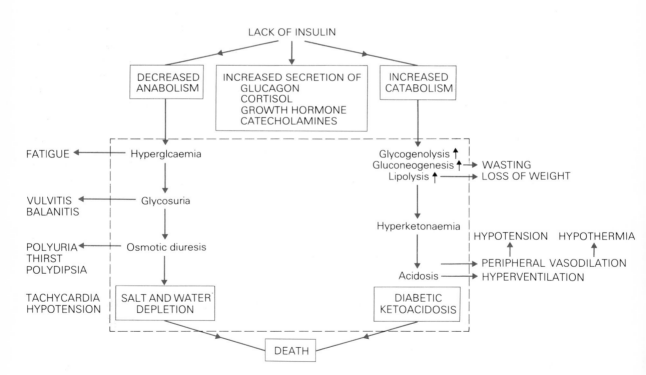

Fig. 8.34 *Pathophysiological basis of the symptoms and signs of untreated or uncontrolled diabetes mellitus.*

pathy, or ulceration of the feet due to a combination of neuropathy, peripheral vascular disease and infection. Uncontrolled diabetes is associated with an increased susceptibility to infection and patients may present with skin sepsis, intractable and recurrent urinary tract infections, pulmonary tuberculosis or poor healing of a wound following surgery.

A minority of cases of diabetes may first present as severe ketoacidosis, either associated with an acute infection or other illness or even without evidence of a precipitating cause. In such cases, abdominal pain and vomiting may be the presenting complaints. This is more likely to occur in IDDM.

Clinical Features

IDDM usually develops during the first 40 years of life in patients of normal or low weight (Fig. 8.32). The majority develop severe symptoms of diabetes acutely over a period of weeks rather than months and, if treatment with insulin is withheld, they rapidly develop fatal ketoacidosis. Such patients usually show no physical signs attributable to the disease. In the fulminating case the most striking features are those of water and salt depletion, that is a loose, dry skin which lifts in folds, a dry, furred tongue and cracked lips, tachycardia, hypotension and reduced intra-ocular pressure. Breathing may be deep and sighing due to acidosis, the breath is usually fetid and the sickly sweet smell of acetone may be apparent. Mental apathy, confusion or coma may also be present.

NIDDM usually appears in middle-aged or elderly patients (Fig. 8.32), most of whom are or have been obese (Fig. 8.29). Such patients are less prone to develop ketoacidosis and in this sense the disease is less severe than IDDM. However, the complications associated with chronic diabetes occur in both clinical types and are more likely to be present in patients with NIDDM at presentation. The physical signs vary depending on the mode of presentation. Pruritus vulvae or balanitis is a common presenting symptom since the external genitalia are especially prone to infection by fungi (Candida) which flourish on skin and mucous membranes contaminated by glucose. Ophthalmoscopy may show the typical appearances of diabetic retinopathy. Depression or loss of the tendon reflexes at the ankles and impaired perception of vibration sensation distally in the legs indicate neuropathy; other abnormalities on neurological examination are less common. The presence of diabetic nephropathy may be indicated by proteinuria in addition to glycosuria. Signs of atherosclerosis are common and may include hypertension, diminished or impalpable pulses in the feet, bruits over the carotid or femoral arteries, and gangrene of the feet. The signs of water and salt depletion with associated mental changes may be seen in cases with severe hyperglycaemia but ketoacidosis is less common (p. 182) so that hyperventilation and a smell of acetone on the breath are unusual.

DIAGNOSIS OF DIABETES

By definition, hyperglycaemia is essential for the diagnosis. When the symptoms suggest diabetes the diagnosis may be confirmed by finding glycosuria, with or without ketonuria, and a random blood glucose concentration greater than 14.0 mmol/l. However, in some cases, particularly those with NIDDM (who have few if any symptoms) and where glycosuria may have been discovered by chance, the diagnosis is more difficult and requires a glucose tolerance test.

The WHO Expert Committee on Diabetes (1985) recommended that a 75-g glucose load should be given orally and that the concentrations of glucose in venous whole blood shown in Table 8.8, should be accepted as normal or diabetic respectively. Values for plasma glucose are about 15% higher than those for whole blood. Intermediate values ('Impaired Glucose Tolerance') call for further evaluation of the patient with a particular attention being directed towards the past medical, obstetric and family history.

Screening

Testing the urine for sugar is the most usual procedure for detecting diabetes, both in the consulting room and in population surveys. Sensitive and glucose-specific dipstick methods are available. A positive response gives a rough indication that the urinary glucose concentration exceeds 0.55–1.11 mmol/l. Semiquantitative measurement of urinary reducing activity can be obtained using copper reduction methods, most conveniently with the Clinitest tablet test. Clinitest tablets and Benedict's reagent are also reduced by other substances in the urine (e.g. lactose, pentose, fructose and galactose) and it may be necessary to identify these by special methods.

If possible the test for urinary glucose should be performed on urine passed $1\frac{1}{2}$–2 hours after a main meal since this will detect more of the milder cases of diabetes than a fasting urine specimen.

The most serious disadvantage of using urinary glucose as a screening procedure is the individual variation in renal threshold; on the one hand, some undoubtedly diabetic individuals will have a negative urine test and, on the other hand, non-diabetic individuals with a low renal threshold for glucose will give a positive result. Wherever practicable, therefore, estimation of the blood glucose concentration two hours after 75 g glucose orally should be used as the screening procedure for detecting diabetes.

In summary, testing the urine for sugar is an essential part of a routine clinical examination. All patients with glycosuria should be considered to be diabetic until proved otherwise on the basis of blood glucose measurements. Particular attention should be paid to high-risk groups, e.g. first-degree relatives of known diabetics, the obese and pregnant women.

The term 'gestational diabetes' is used to refer to the hyperglycaemia which can occur temporarily during pregnancy in individuals who have an inherited liability to develop diabetes. Normal pregnancy is character-ised by hyperinsulinaemia in response to the produc-tion of insulin antagonists such as human placental lactogen (HPL) and progesterone. A suboptimal endo-crine pancreas may be unable to meet this demand. Since even minimal hyperglycaemia in pregnancy is associated with an increased fetal loss (p. 194), it is important to detect and treat these cases effectively. Detection may present problems since glycosuria is common in normal pregnancy (due to a fall in the renal threshold for glucose secondary to an increase in the glomerular filtration rate) and in late pregnancy through lactose appearing in the urine. The finding of reducing substances in the urine of a pregnant woman should, however, never be lightly dismissed and in all cases the blood glucose concentration should be carefully mea-sured (using an assay specific for glucose) in the fasting state and at accurately-timed intervals after a 75-g glucose load. The diagnostic criteria for diabetes in pregnancy are more stringent than those recom-mended for non-pregnant subjects and those with Impaired Glucose Tolerance should be treated as diabetic.

TREATMENT OF DIABETES

Three methods of treatment are available: diet alone; diet and an oral hypoglycaemic drug; and diet and insulin. Approximately 50% of new cases of diabetes can be controlled adequately by diet alone, about 30% will need an oral hypoglycaemic drug, and 20% will require insulin. The age and the weight of the patient at diagnosis indicate with a high degree of probability the type of treatment likely to be required (Fig. 8.35) but the regimen eventually adopted in each individual case is ultimately chosen by a process of clinical trial.

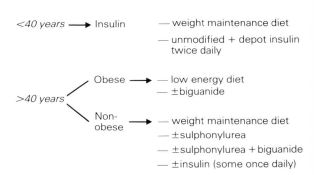

Fig. 8.35 *The long-term type of treatment probably required by any individual patient can be determined by considering his age and weight at diagnosis of diabetes.*

Dietary Treatment: General Principles

Satisfactory treatment of all diabetic patients involves some dietary restriction.

The first step in preparing any dietary regimen is to decide what the individual patient's daily *energy* requirement is. This must be estimated after consider-ing such factors as age, sex, actual weight in relation to desirable weight, activity, occupation and financial resources. An approximate range for the various groups of patients might be: 1. an obese, middle-aged or elderly patient, 1000–1600 kcal daily; 2. an elderly diabetic not overweight, 1400–1800 kcal daily; 3. a young, active diabetic, 1800–3000 kcal daily. The body weight should be maintained at or slightly below the ideal for the patient's height. Thus the range for group 2 may have to be extended if it is not sufficient to maintain weight, and young overweight patients in group 3 may have their daily intake reduced to below 1800 kcal.

Next, the proportion of energy derived from carbohydrate, protein and fat must be allocated. The approximate ratio in the British national diet is: protein 12%, fat 42% and carbohydrate 46%. A high proportion of the fat intake is saturated, and much of the carbohydrate is refined, i.e. sucrose. This type of diet is generally considered to be atherogenic, and diabetic patients are peculiarly susceptible to atherosclerosis (p. 184). Therefore it is recommended that the energy derived from fat should be reduced to about 30–35% and that from carbohydrate and protein increased to 50–55% and 15% respectively.

All the *carbohydrate* prescribed should be in the form of starch. Readily-absorbed carbohydrates (e.g. glucose and sucrose) should generally be avoided because they produce a sudden rise in the blood glucose concentration. The daily intake of carbohydrate ranges from 100 g (the minimum sufficient to prevent ketonuria) to a maximum of 280 g (the highest at which satisfactory blood glucose levels can usually be maintained). If total carbohydrate intake is 240 g per day, each of three main meals can provide 50 g, three snacks provide 60 g, and 30 g comes in 0.5 l milk taken in the course of the day. It is difficult to prevent an excessive rise in blood glucose after each meal with larger amounts of carbohydrate at a sitting.

Protein consumption is determined largely by social and economic considerations and may sometimes be relatively low. Every effort should be made to ensure that some protein-rich food is eaten at each meal. There are two reasons for this. Firstly, in NIDDM a high intake of protein will increase the secretion of insulin and help to compensate for the defect in glucose-mediated insulin secretion seen in so many of these patients. Secondly, protein promotes satiety and helps both categories of patient to adhere to the carbohydrate allowance. Protein consumption will usually be 60–110 g per day.

Fat consumption should be adjusted to bring the total energy intake to the desired level; it usually amounts to 50–150 g per day. The proportion of unsaturated fat should be increased if possible. Plasma lipids should be checked regularly and, if significantly elevated, the diet may be further modified.

A high intake of *fibre* will increase satiety and reduce constipation, and may help to lower the plasma concentration of lipid and glucose.

There is no medical objection to diabetic patients taking alcoholic drinks in moderation provided that the patient appreciates that account must be taken of their energy and sometimes of their carbohydrate content.

Types of Diet

Two basic types of diet are used in the treatment of diabetes: low energy, weight-reducing diets and weight-maintenance diets.

Weight-reducing diets

The benefits of reduction in body weight on the metabolism of the obese patient with NIDDM are well documented. Even where the initial blood glucose concentration is high and the plasma immunoreactive insulin low, additional treatment with insulin or an oral hypoglycaemic agent can often be avoided (Fig. 8.36). The benefit of weight reduction on the mortality rate of obese non-diabetic persons is well known, and applies even more strikingly to obese diabetics. The precise mechanism of this effect is uncertain. Treatment of obese people, both diabetic and non-diabetic, with a diet low in refined and high in unrefined carbohydrate, and restricted in total energy content, results in an increased number of insulin receptors on adipocytes which is associated with a rapid fall in the blood glucose concentration in diabetic subjects. Reduction in body weight increases this effect and, in the long term, the plasma insulin concentration rises in many (though not all) patients.

Weight-maintenance diabetic diets

Dietary measures are an essential part of the treatment

Obese diabetic

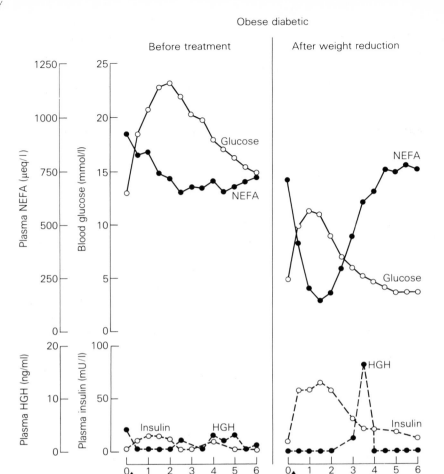

Fig. 8.36 *Changes in the concentration of blood glucose and plasma non-esterified fatty acids, immunoreactive insulin, and human growth hormone following ingestion of 50 g glucose (↑) in an obese patient with NIDDM at diagnosis and after reduction in weight. Note the marked rise in plasma IRI and the restoration of the normal postabsorptive surge of HGH following treatment with a low energy diet.*

of diabetic patients who require treatment with an oral hypoglycaemic drug or insulin. By adjusting the amount and the time of the intake of food, particularly the amount of carbohydrate, and the dose of insulin or oral hypoglycaemic agent, an attempt is made to keep the fluctuation in blood glucose concentration to a minimum and as near as possible to the normal range. If the intake of food varies from day to day it is impossible to devise a reasonably steady insulin or other regime to

cover it. If a fixed daily intake is to be achieved and monotony avoided an exchange system is necessary. The 'exchanges' or portions employed as units are arbitrary, decided mainly on the basis of the food habits of the population as a whole. In most parts of the world the carbohydrate unit recommended is 10 g. In Britain the staple carbohydrate food is bread, and the basic carbohydrate exchange for the purposes of calculation is 20 g bread, which contains 10 g carbohydrate. When the patient's requirements have been assessed the figures must be translated into practical instructions in the form of a diet sheet. Each patient has a list of 10-g carbohydrate portions and the number of portions to be taken at each time of the day is specified.

Oral Hypoglycaemic Drugs

A number of compounds are effective in reducing hyperglycaemia in patients who would otherwise require insulin. These drugs fall into two categories: the sulphonylureas and the biguanides. Although their mechanism of action is different, the effect of both groups of drugs depends upon a supply of endogenous insulin and they therefore have no hypoglycaemic effect in patients with IDDM.

Sulphonylureas

Mechanism of action: The initial effect of sulphonylurea compounds in lowering blood glucose concentration is due to stimulation of the release of insulin from the pancreatic B cell. The long-term hypoglycaemic effect, however, seems to be due to extrapancreatic effects, particularly in reducing the hepatic release of glucose and insulin resistance.

Indications for use: Sulphonylureas are valuable in the treatment of non-obese NIDDM patients who fail to respond to simple dietary restriction. Although sulphonylureas will lower the blood glucose concentration of obese NIDDM patients such patients should be treated energetically by dietary restriction and weight reduction, since the sulphonylureas tend to promote an increase in weight and in the long run this will intensify the total disability. Only if it is clear that dietary measures alone are inadequate should patients be started on an oral hypoglycaemic drug.

Table 8.13 lists the sulphonylureas in common use. The main difference between the individual compounds is their length of action.

Table 8.13
Sulphonylureas – Comparative Features

Official name	Tablet size (mg)	Range of dose (mg)	Potency	Approximate biological half-life (h)	Particular aspects
Acetohexamide	500	500–1500	Medium	5	
Chlorpropamide	{ 100 250	100–500	Strong	40	Flushing after alcohol, occasional cholestatic jaundice
Glibenclamide	5	2.5–20	Strong and quick	12	May provoke severe hypoglycaemia, particularly in the elderly
Glibornuride	25	12.5–75	Strong	8	
Glipizide	5	2.5–30	Strong	3.5	
Glymidine	500	500–2000	Medium	4	A sulphapyrimidine with virtually no cross-reaction with sulphonylureas in regard to skin rashes
Tolazamide	{ 100 250	100–750	Strong	7	
Tolbutamide	500	500–3000	Relatively weak	4	Metabolite gives flaky precipitate with sulpho-salicylic acid or picric acid (Esbach's reagent) or when acidified and boiled; hence false positive tests for proteinuria (not with Albustix)

Tolbutamide is the mildest and probably also the safest of the sulphonylureas. It is very well tolerated and toxic reactions occur only rarely. Its duration of action is relatively short so that it has to be given two or three times daily. Tolbutamide is a useful drug in the elderly where the risk and the consequences of inducing hypoglycaemia are increased.

Chlorpropamide has a bioligical half-life of about 36 hours and an effective concentration can be maintained in the blood by a single dose at breakfast. The usual maintenance dose is between 100 and 350 mg daily; larger doses should not be used on a long-term basis since above this level there is an increased risk of toxic effects such as jaundice, rashes and blood dyscrasia. Facial flushing after taking alcohol occurs in some patients. This reaction can be blocked with naloxone, which suggests that in these patients the flush may be related to endorphins.

Chlorpropamide may lead to severe hypoglycaemia which can be refractory to treatment. Care must be taken to avoid this, particularly in elderly patients, and once glycosuria has been abolished and symptoms relieved the daily dose of chlorpropamide should be reduced to the minimum required to maintain control. Many patients requiring 250–350 mg daily initially can be maintained on a long-term basis on 100 mg per day.

Other sulphonylureas such as acetohexamide, tolazamide, glibenclamide, glipizide and glymidine are more expensive and usually offer little advantage over tolbutamide and chlorpropamide but may be useful in individual patients.

Biguanides

The biguanides metformin and phenformin are less widely used in Britain than the sulphonylureas because of the higher incidence of side-effects, particularly gastrointestinal symptoms, and because there has been a significant number of deaths from lactic acidosis in patients taking these drugs, particularly phenformin.

Mechanism of action: The mechanism of action of these compounds has not been precisely defined. They have no hypoglycaemic effect in normal people but, in the diabetic, insulin sensitivity and peripheral glucose uptake are increased. There is some evidence that they also impair glucose absorption and reduce hepatic

gluconeogenesis. Despite their effect in lowering the blood glucose level in diabetic patients, hypoglycaemia does not occur in patients taking these compounds.

Indications for use: Despite its disadvantages, metformin may be useful in two difficult clinical situations. Firstly, its administration is not associated with a rise in body weight, and it may therefore be preferred when an obese patient with NIDDM must be treated because hyperglycaemia persists despite efforts to adhere to a diet or reduce weight. Secondly, as the hypoglycaemic effect of the biguanides appears to be synergistic with that of the sulphonylureas, there is a place for combining the two drugs when the sulphonylureas alone have proved inadequate and when, as happens in 5–10% of patients, initial success is followed after several months or years by loss of control, i.e. when 'secondary failure' occurs. Such combined therapy should be used, however, only when there are clear contraindications to treatment with insulin since, despite euglycaemia, the plasma concentration of intermediary metabolites (including lactate, pyruvate, alanine, glycerol and ketone bodies) is abnormal in patients treated in this way.

Metformin is given with food two or three times daily. Its use is contra-indicated in patients with impaired renal or hepatic function and in those who take alcohol in excess because the risk of lactic acidosis is significantly increased in such patients. Its administration should be discontinued, at least temporarily, if any other serious medical condition develops; treatment with insulin is then substituted.

The increased blood lactate levels seen in patients taking biguanides seem to result from an increased flow of glucose through glycolysis combined with reduced lactate removal due, partly at least, to inhibition of gluconeogenesis.

Insulin

Conventional methods of treatment have relied upon subcutaneous injection of insulin extracted from the pancreas of cattle and pigs. A crude attempt is made to imitate the responsiveness of the normal B cell to ingestion of nutrients by insulin regimens combining unmodified (quick and short-acting) insulin with depot (slow and long-acting) insulin. By regulating the quan-

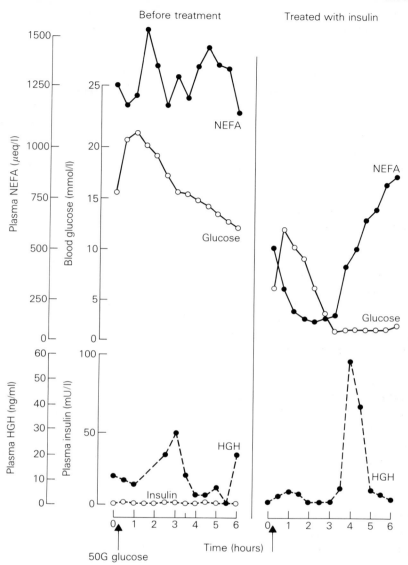

Fig. 8.37 *Changes in the concentration of blood glucose and plasma non-esterified fatty acids, immunoreactive insulin, and human growth hormone following ingestion of 50 g glucose in* a thin patient with IDDM at diagnosis and after treatment with insulin. Note the restoration of normal metabolism (comparable to that seen in Fig. 8.10) after treatment with insulin.

tity and timing of the food eaten, particularly carbohydrate, and dovetailing the dose of insulin, an attempt is made to achieve a normal, flat, daily profile of glycaemia throughout the day and night.

Although intensive treatment with insulin diminishes the post-receptor defect and rapidly restores the metabolism to normal (Fig. 8.37), in many, if not most, established cases of IDDM, control of the blood glucose is far from normal even in the early stages of the disease (Fig. 8.38). Factors contributing to instability of the blood glucose include variations in the amount of exercise taken, in the rate at which various foods release their carbohydrate products of digestion, in the rate at which insulin is absorbed into the bloodstream at different sites in the body, and in the quantity and type of circulating insulin-binding antibodies.

For many years insulin was regarded as non-antigenic. In 1956 Berson and Yalow demonstrated that the serum of diabetic patients treated with exogenous insulin contained immunoglobulins which could bind insulin. This led them to develop radioimmunological methods for the assay of hormones in plasma. They were awarded a Nobel Prize for this work.

It is now known that even homologous pancreatic

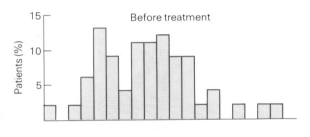

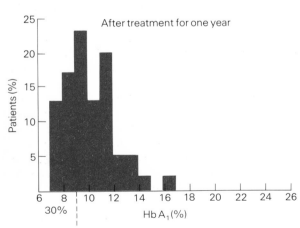

Fig. 8.38 *Distribution of glycosylated haemoglobin (HbA₁) concentration in consecutive patients referred with IDDM to the Diabetic Clinic, Western General Hospital, Edinburgh, before and after treatment for one year. The normal range is 6–8%. A value of 9% or less was considered satisfactory. Only 30% achieved this.*

insulin can, in some circumstances, act as a weak antigen. The degree of antigenicity of therapeutic preparations of insulin in man is related to several factors such as its animal source, physical properties and most importantly its purity. Thus greater antigenicity is shown by preparations of bovine than porcine insulin (which differs from human insulin in respect of only one amino acid), by an acid rather than a neutral solution of insulin, and by preparations containing polypeptide molecules other than insulin, whether these are deliberately added (depot insulins) or present as contaminants.

The older preparations of insulin are thus strongly antigenic because they usually consist of bovine insulin, are commonly prepared at low pH, frequently contain added protein to delay their action, and always contain proinsulin and pancreatic hormones other than insulin. Studies of patients with long-standing IDDM being treated with conventional insulin have shown insulin-binding antibodies in 100% of patients and circulating antibodies to human pancreatic polypeptides in 63%, to vasoactive intestinal peptide in 6%, to glucagon in 6%, and to somatostatin in 0.5%. Immunocytochemical testing shows antibody-positive diabetic plasma reacting specifically against the corresponding hormone-producing cells in the endocrine pancreas, enteroglucagon and somatostatin-producing cells outside the pancreas, and against VIP-containing autonomic nerves throughout the body, i.e. 'iatrogenic autoimmunity' to naturally-occurring hormones. Whether this causes adverse effects on the action of these hormones and the tissues which produce them is unknown, but the presence of circulating insulin-binding antibodies undoubtedly has several well-defined consequences.

For example: 1. At a given dose of insulin, in the presence of antibodies, the increase in plasma-free insulin is sluggish, peak concentrations are lower and delayed and, because the half-life of insulin is prolonged, persistent hyperinsulinaemia may occur. High-affinity antibodies can compete with receptors for insulin, whereas high-capacity antibodies can serve as a reservoir for insulin and, although it has been suggested that these may act as a stabilising factor, insulin may 'leak' off these antibodies at inappropriate times, causing unexpected hypoglycaemia.

2. Assay of plasma C-peptide in patients with treated IDDM has shown that almost all retain some residual B cell function in the first two years of diabetes. Thereafter the percentage with detectable plasma C-peptide falls steadily with the duration of the diabetes. Residual B cell function appears to

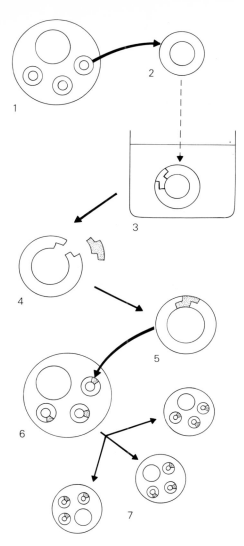

Fig. 8.39 *Diagrammatic representation of the principles of the method for synthesising insulin by recombinant DNA technology. (1) An E. Coli bacterium containing a single chromosome and several small rings of genetic material (plasmids). (2) After breaking open the bacterium with detergent the plasmids are isolated by centrifugation and (3) immersed in a restriction enzyme causing them to open at a specific place on the ring. (4) The insulin gene is then spliced into the bacterium's plasmids, thus forming 'recombinant DNA' (5). (6) The hybrid plasmids are reinserted into a bacterium. (7) The cell divides, replicating all its genes, including the new DNA.*

favour stability in IDDM. There is evidence that insulin-binding antibodies may adversely influence B cell function in IDDM.

3. It has been shown that insulin-binding antibodies cross the placenta and are deposited in various fetal organs including the pancreas. Certain changes (including lymphocytic infiltration and fibrosis) can also be seen in the pancreas of infants born to mothers with IDDM. It has been suggested that these might predispose to the subsequent development of diabetes.

4. High immunogenicity increases the incidence of the insulin resistance, generalised insulin allergy and localised atrophy at injection sites.

Use of 'monocomponent' pig insulins (purified by ion exchange chromatography) has abolished 'iatrogenic autoimmunity', reduced the incidence of insulin resistance, generalised insulin allergy and localised fat atrophy, and diminished the formation of insulin-binding antibodies to negligible levels in most patients.

The production of human insulin by recombinant DNA technology (Fig. 8.39) represents a major scientific achievement. Nevertheless there is as yet little evidence to suggest that there are major (or even minor) clinical differences between biosynthetic human insulin and purified pork insulin.

Clinical use of insulin

The treatment of diabetes mellitus with insulin became possible only because of the development of accurate methods of standardisation. The dose is measured in units, each representing a degree of hypoglycaemic activity. This was first defined in 1922 by Banting and Best and was based on the ability of samples of insulin to lower the blood glucose concentration in rabbits. In 1925, the unit of insulin was defined by reference to a standard preparation with an activity of approximately 24 U/mg. Today insulin is assayed by comparing it with the Fourth International Standard Insulin Preparation (1958) in its effect on lowering the blood glucose concentration of mice to a lethal level. Therapeutic preparations of insulin usually contain 20, 40, 80 or 100 U/ml.

There are two main types of insulin in clinical use: unmodified, rapid onset, short-acting; and modified or 'depot', delayed onset, long-acting preparations (Table 8.14). Unmodified insulins are clear solutions which, when injected subcutaneously, produce an effect in about 30 minutes which lasts for approximately 6 hours. Unmodified insulin is essential in new cases of

Table 8.14

Main Types of Preparations of Insulin and Duration of Action

Type	Examples of proprietary preparations in common use		Species	Approx. duration of action (hours)
Rapid/Short − Unmodified				6
Soluble or regular insulin (acid)	Soluble insulin	(Wellcome)	Cattle	
Neutral insulins	Neusulin	(Wellcome)	Cattle	
	Velosulin	(Nordisk)	Pig	
	Humulin S	(Eli Lilly)	Human (biosynthetic)	
	Actrapid MC	(Novo)	Pig	
	Actrapid HM	(Novo)	Human (semisynthetic)	
Intermediate − Modified − Depot				12
Isophane type insulins	Neuphane	(Wellcome)	Cattle	
	Insulatard	(Nordisk)	Pig	
	Humulin I	(Eli Lilly)	Human (biosynthetic)	
Insulin zinc suspensions	Monotard MC	(Novo)	Pig	
	Protophane HM	(Novo)	Human (semisynthetic)	
Slow/Long − Modified − Depot				
Isophane type insulin	Humulin Zn	(Eli Lilly)	Human (biosynthetic)	16 +
Insulin zinc suspensions	Ultratard MC	(Novo)	Pig	24 +
	Ultratard HM	(Novo)	Human (semisynthetic)	

All these insulins are available in highly purified form and in three strengths, i.e. 40, 80 and 100 international units/ml. Soluble insulin is also available as a solution containing 20 iu/ml. In the UK and USA U100 insulin only is available for routine clinical use.

diabetes with severe dehydration and/or ketoacidosis, in acute metabolic decompensation in established cases of diabetes (both ID and NID) from whatever cause, in combination with depot insulins for the day-to-day management of nearly all young patients with diabetes, and in any situation where intravenous insulin is required, for example in infusion pumps.

Depot insulin preparations are cloudy solutions. Their delayed and prolonged action can be achieved in two main ways. In isophane preparations, insulin is adsorbed on to a foreign protein molecule, protamine, in the presence of zinc; when injected subcutaneously, the protein-zinc-insulin complex breaks up slowly in the tissues, gradually releasing the bound insulin over a period of 12–24 hours. Insulin zinc suspensions do not contain foreign protein. The duration of their action depends on the size and form of the insulin crystals as well as on the rate at which these crystals are dissolved and absorbed. The former is achieved by carefully controlling the conditions of precipitation; the latter is delayed by buffering with acetate and by adding small quantities of zinc. In a few elderly patients satisfactory control can be established by a single morning injection of depot insulin. Most IDDM patients, however, do best by taking unmodified insulin along with one of the intermediate depot insulins before breakfast and repeating this combination before the evening meal.

Examples of suitable commercial preparations are listed in Table 8.14.

In practice, various combinations of the numerous available insulin preparations can be tried and the time at which they are administered altered on the basis of the results of blood glucose estimations at different times of the day until good metabolic control is achieved over 24 hours. It is impossible to forecast the response of a patient to insulin and the daily dose required to establish satisfactory control varies widely and is established by clinical trial.

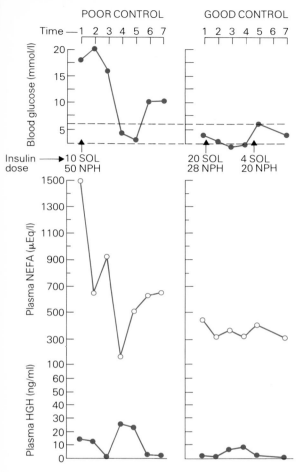

POOR CONTROL   GOOD CONTROL

Time —1 2 3 4 5 6 7   1 2 3 4 5 6 7

Blood glucose (mmol/l)

Insulin → 10 SOL   20 SOL   4 SOL
dose   50 NPH   28 NPH   20 NPH

Plasma NEFA (μEq/l)

Plasma HGH (ng/ml)

Fig. 8.40 *Blood glucose and plasma non-esterified fatty acids (1) fasting, (2) 1½ hours after breakfast, (3) and (4) before and 1½ hours after the midday meal, (5) and (6) before and 1½ hours after the evening meal, and (7) before going to bed, in a non-obese, 14-year-old girl with IDDM, undertaking normal activity in the course of the day. Diabetes had been diagnosed 11 years previously and she was following a diet of 9.2 MJ distributed in three main meals and three snacks taken at mid-morning, mid-afternoon and bedtime. Her diabetes was poorly controlled by 60 units of insulin taken in a single daily dose before breakfast. Greatly improved control was achieved by a slight increase in the total daily amount of insulin given and by administering this in two doses. The broken lines in the upper panel indicate the physiological range for the blood glucose concentration.*

Factors determining the type and amount of insulin required in an individual case include the patient's sensitivity to the action of insulin (thin subjects are generally more sensitive than the obese) and way of life, e.g. meal pattern, occupation and hours of work, and the amount and timing of exercise. More insulin will be needed to cover main meals and periods of inactivity, and vice versa. Figure 8.40 shows an example of a patient poorly controlled by one insulin regime but well controlled by another.

Patient Education

All insulin-requiring patients who are capable of doing so must learn to measure their dose of insulin accurately with an insulin syringe, to manage their own injections and to adjust the dose themselves on the basis of urinary and/or blood glucose measurements and other factors such as illness, unusual exercise and insulin-induced hypoglycaemic episodes. They must therefore have a working knowledge of diabetes and must have ready access to medical advice should the need arise. This education is time-consuming but it is the only way that patients can safely undertake all normal activities while maintaining good metabolic control. If the patient is a child, or an adult who is incapable for whatever reason of coping independently, instructions must be given to a parent or other attendant.

Assessment of Metabolic Control

The aim of treatment is to achieve a normal metabolic state. This will usually be possible if the body weight is maintained near the ideal level and the blood glucose concentration kept constantly within the physiological range.

The various methods of assessing blood glucose control are listed in Table 8.15.

Semiquantitative preprandial urine testing is the time-honoured method of assessing control. This is usually done using Clinitest tablets or Diastix strips. The former method is more inconvenient but is more accurate when glycosuria is severe and particularly when ketonuria is present since this inhibits colour development in the Diastix strip. The Diabur 5000

Table 8.15

Methods of Assessing Blood Glucose Control

Urinary glucose
    preprandial tests
    24 hour collection

Blood glucose
    single, random clinic measurements
    day profiles:
        inpatients
        day patients
    capillary blood spot profiles: home-based patients
    patient home monitoring:
        test-strips (visual)
        test-strips (meters)

Glycosylated proteins
    haemoglobin
    albumin
    total serum proteins (fructosamine)

test-strip avoids these problems. The correlation between tests for urinary glucose and the blood glucose concentration is affected by the length of time the urine has been in the bladder and by the renal threshold for glucose. Even where patients have emptied the bladder half to one hour before passing the specimen to be tested there is a poor correlation between simultaneous urinary and blood glucose estimations (Fig. 8.41).

The overwhelming disadvantage of using the blood glucose concentration as a measure of overall control in the diabetic is its lability. Single random blood glucose estimations obtained at routine clinic visits are therefore of limited value. The main disadvantage of the kind of day profile illustrated in Fig. 8.40 is that it is obtained in a highly artificial situation. The great advantage of the blood spot profile and of home monitoring of blood glucose by patients themselves is that tests are performed in the real-life situation. In the former, patients collect serial capillary blood samples by finger-prick on to filter paper strips previously soaked in boric acid. When the series is complete the strips are posted to the laboratory for estimation. The disadvantage of this system is the delay in obtaining

results. The great advantage of self-monitoring of blood glucose concentration by patients is that information is immediately available and permits well-informed and motivated patients to make appropriate adjustments in insulin and/or diet on a day-to-day basis. Thus serious ketoacidosis is avoided and a normal or near normal metabolism achieved without frequent and disabling

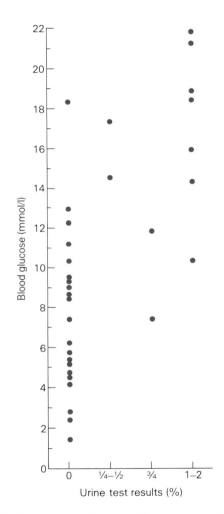

Fig. 8.41 *Simultaneous urinary and blood glucose estimations performed over a two week period in a 14-year-old girl taking twice daily injections of insulin for one year. Note that when the urinary test records 0 the blood glucose concentration ranges from 1.5–18 mmol/l.*

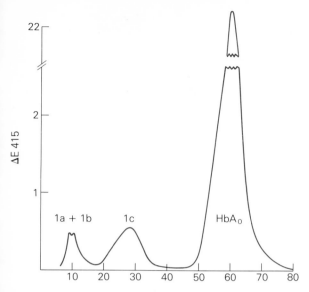

Fig. 8.42 *Elution profile of human haemoglobin from chromatographic column.*

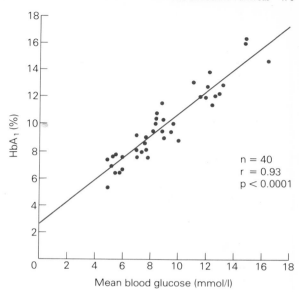

Fig. 8.43 *The relationship between % HbA, and mean blood glucose levels in the previous three months. Each dot represents the mean blood glucose concentration for a single patient. Each patient collected capillary blood samples before and two hours after each main meal for 24 hours every two weeks for three months.*

hypoglycaemia. A range of methods is available, but in all of them a capillary blood sample is placed on an enzyme-impregnated stick (e.g. Dextrostix or BM Glycemie 20–800), and the colour developed is either compared visually with a standard colour chart or, more accurately, read with a simple colorimetric meter.

When haemoglobin from a normal adult is passed through a chromatographic column it separates into the major component haemoglobin A (HbA) comprising 92–94% of the total, and several minor, fast-moving components collectively known as haemoglobin A_1 (HbA_1) comprising 6–8% of the total (Fig. 8.42). These are structurally identical to HbA except for the addition of a glucose group to the terminal amino acid of the beta chain. This is a post-synthetic, non-enzymatic reaction and the rate of synthesis of HbA_1 is a function of the exposure of the red cell to glucose. Since the glucose linkage is relatively stable, HbA_1 accumulates throughout the lifespan of the erythrocyte and its concentration reflects the mean blood glucose concentration over the previous few months. Measurement of HbA_1 can therefore be used as a supplement to blood glucose estimations to monitor the overall degree of

diabetic control achieved. Figure 8.43 shows the close relationship between HbA_1 and the mean blood glucose concentration in 40 patients with IDDM over a three-month period. The very close correlation obtained between HbA_1 and mean blood glucose concentration supports the expectation that such measurements taken during a normal working day are more representative of the usual prevailing blood glucose levels than those obtained in hospital in- or outpatients.

Glycosylation of haemoglobin is just one example of the many glycosylation reactions which occur in the body. Glycosylated serum proteins can also be measured and, because of their shorter half-life, give an indication of glycaemic control over the preceding few weeks rather than months.

Concentration of serum lipids is another important index of overall metabolic control in diabetic patients and should be monitored regularly.

ACUTE COMPLICATIONS OF TREATMENT

Hypoglycaemia

If unmodified insulin is administered to a normal person the blood glucose falls; symptoms usually begin to appear when the concentration is about 2.7 mmol/l and are fully developed at about 2.2 mmol/l. These may include any of the following: a feeling of weakness and emptiness, hunger, sweating, palpitations, tremulousness, faintness, dizziness, headache, diplopia and mental confusion. Abnormal behaviour, characterised particularly by aggression and poor coordination, is common and may be mistaken for drunkenness. Alternatively, and particularly in children, there may be lassitude and somnolence or muscular twitchings. Eventually coma, sometimes with convulsions, may follow.

Hypoglycaemia induces secretion of adrenaline (p. 156) which raises the blood glucose concentration by increasing glycogenolysis and is responsible for inducing some of the classical clinical features of hypoglycaemia, i.e. pallor, palpitations, tachycardia and tremor. This homeostatic mechanism partly explains why patients rarely die of hypoglycaemic coma from too much unmodified insulin. By contrast, coma is likely to be more severe and dangerous when it occurs as a result of an overdose of depot insulin or a long-acting sulphonylurea such as chlorpropamide. Since the brain is glucose-dependent metabolically, permanent brain damage may result from prolonged hypoglycaemia.

Hypoglycaemia due to overdosage with unmodified insulin is liable to occur at the time when the insulin has its maximum effect – morning or early evening – and usually elicits classical symptoms and responds rapidly to treatment. Hypoglycaemia from excessive depot insulin given before breakfast usually occurs in the late afternoon, while depot insulin given before the evening meal is responsible for hypoglycaemia developing through the night into the early hours of the morning. In this case the fall in blood glucose concentration may be more gradual and elicit little adrenaline response, become persistent and profound and respond more slowly to treatment. The predominant warning symptoms, which are very variable, include headache, night sweats, nausea leading sometimes to troublesome vomiting, mental confusion

and drowsiness, especially before breakfast.

The incidence of nocturnal hypoglycaemia in IDDM patients treated conventionally is difficult to establish. It is certainly a common problem when attempts are made to achieve a normal or near normal blood glucose concentration throughout 24 hours. The basic cause is the physiological variation in the amount of insulin required to achieve homeostasis (Table 8.16) which is probably related to the diurnal variation in the secretion of anti-insulin hormones such as cortisol and growth hormone. Thus there is a tendency for hypoglycaemia at 0300 hours combined with hyperglycaemia at 0800. This is compounded by the quicker, shorter action of the highly purified depot insulins so that intermediate preparations are likely to exert their maximum action at 0300 hours (when the insulin requirement is lowest) and vice versa. This problem can be dealt with effectively by splitting the evening dose, with unmodified insulin only before the evening meal and the evening depot insulin taken at bedtime. Alternatively, the disadvantage of having to take three daily injections can sometimes be overcome by substituting a long depot insulin (e.g. Ultratard) for the more usual intermediate preparation before the evening meal.

Table 8.16
Nocturnal Hypoglycaemia in IDDM

Incidence ?

Cause:
  i. variation in overnight insulin requirement
     2400–0400 8 mU/kg/h
     0400–0800 16 mU/kg/h
  ii. quicker, shorter action of highly purified depot insulins compared with older insulins with greater immunogenicity

Diagnosis:
  accurate blood glucose estimations at 0300 *and* 0800

Treatment:
  adjust insulin regimen
  either split evening dose
  or use long depot insulin (e.g. Ultratard) before evening meal instead of intermediate preparation

Exercise and hypoglycaemia

Figure 8.44 shows that the effect of exercise in treated IDDM depends on the prevailing metabolic state. On the one hand, well-controlled patients are invariably hyperinsulinaemic so that during exercise increased peripheral glucose uptake is not compensated for by increased hepatic release of glucose (as is normal, Fig. 8.23) and hypoglycaemia occurs; on the other hand poorly-controlled patients are relatively hypo-insulinaemic and exercise may aggravate hyperglycaemia and ketonaemia.

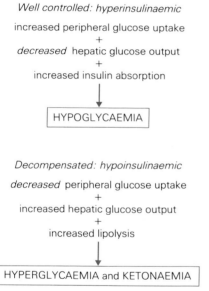

Well controlled: hyperinsulinaemic

increased peripheral glucose uptake
+
decreased hepatic glucose output
+
increased insulin absorption
↓
HYPOGLYCAEMIA

Decompensated: hypoinsulinaemic

decreased peripheral glucose uptake
+
increased hepatic glucose output
+
increased lipolysis
↓
HYPERGLYCAEMIA and KETONAEMIA

Fig. 8.44 *The effect of exercise in diabetic patients being treated with insulin.*

Causes and prevention

The most common causes of hypoglycaemia in patients taking insulin or a sulphonylurea are unpunctual meals and unaccustomed exercise. Both causes are avoidable. The preceding dose of insulin should be reduced appropriately if unusual activity is anticipated, and extra carbohydrate may also be required. Diabetic patients should experience hypoglycaemia under

Table 8.17

Patients with IDDM May Have Problems Associated with Insulin-induced Hypoglycaemia

1. *Impaired recovery from insulin-induced hypoglycaemia due to*
   (a) glucagon response   ↓
   (b) catecholamine response   ↓
   (c) plasma free insulin   ↑

2. *Post-hypoglycaemic hyperglycaemia due to*
   (a) sympatho-adrenal activation
            +
   (b) insulin deficiency

3. *Loss of symptoms of hypoglycaemia*

supervision so that they can learn to recognise the early symptoms. They should always carry some tablets of glucose or lumps of sugar for use in an emergency.

Patients with long-standing IDDM may have particular problems associated with insulin-induced hypoglycaemia (Table 8.17). In many such patients the mechanisms which correct insulin-induced hypoglycaemia in normal people (Fig. 8.25) are defective. In particular, sympathetic neuropathy (p. 194) may result in the loss of both the glucagon and catecholamine response to hypoglycaemia so that glucose recovery fails to occur. There is also evidence that those who experience recurrent hypoglycaemia may develop hypothalamic dysfunction.

Post-hypoglycaemic hyperglycaemia is particularly common before breakfast. This phenomenon (first described by Somogyi) will not occur unless there is absolute or relative deficiency of insulin. Note that impaired recovery from insulin-induced hypoglycaemia and post-hypoglycaemic hyperglycaemia will not coexist.

A further problem for many long-standing IDD patients is loss of symptoms of hypoglycaemia which is also usually due to sympathetic neuropathy. Home blood glucose monitoring is mandatory in these patients and their relatives should be instructed in the use of glucagon as described below.

Treatment of hypoglycaemic episodes

If recognised early, hypoglycaemia may be corrected

easily by ingestion of carbohydrate, preferably in an easily absorbable form.

If patients are so stuporous that they cannot swallow, a subcutaneous or intramuscular injection of 1 mg glucagon may be given, repeated if necessary after 10 minutes. The hyperglycaemic effect is transitory so that carbohydrate must be ingested as soon as the patient recovers consciousness. Glucagon may not be effective in severe and prolonged hypoglycaemia due to depot insulins, when intravenous glucose may be required.

Diabetic Ketoacidosis

Prior to the discovery of insulin, more than 50% of diabetic patients died of ketoacidosis. Today this complication should account for less than 2% of deaths in diabetics. However, in some parts of the world both the incidence and the mortality from diabetic ketoacidosis are much higher. Its prevention is largely a matter of education of both patients and doctors. A significant number of new patients still present in diabetic ketoacidosis and, in established diabetics, a common course of events is that patients develop an intercurrent infection, lose their appetite, and either stop or drastically reduce their dose of insulin (on either their own initiative or their doctor's advice) in the mistaken belief that under these circumstances less insulin is required. Any form of stress, particularly that produced by infection, may precipitate severe ketoacidosis in even the mildest case of diabetes. In a significant proportion of cases the precipitating cause cannot be identified.

A clear understanding of the biochemical basis and pathophysiology of this disorder (p. 166) is essential for its efficient treatment. Hyperglycaemia and ketoacidosis are not always necessarily closely correlated. Even moderate hyperglycaemia may be associated with life-threatening acidosis, particularly in young patients with IDDM, while coma can occur, usually in elderly patients, with extreme hyperglycaemia and dehydration but no ketoacidosis. This is known as *hyperosmolar diabetic coma.*

Table 8.18 shows the average loss of fluid and electrolytes in moderately severe diabetic ketoacidosis in an adult. About half of the deficit of total body water is derived from the intracellular compartment and

Table 8.18

Average Loss of Fluid and Electrolytes in an Adult with Diabetic Ketoacidosis of Moderate Severity

Water:	6 litres
Sodium:	500 mmol
Chloride:	400 mmol
Potassium:	350+ mmol

occurs comparatively early in the development of acidosis with relatively few clinical features; the remainder represents loss of extracellular fluid sustained largely in the later stages. It is at this time that marked contraction of the size of the extracellular space occurs, with haemoconcentration, a decrease in blood volume, and finally a fall in blood pressure with associated renal ischaemia and oliguria.

Every patient in diabetic ketoacidosis is potassium-depleted, but the plasma concentrations of potassium and sodium give very little indication of total body deficit. They may even be raised initially due to disproportionate loss of water and catabolism of protein and glycogen. However, soon after treatment with insulin is started there is likely to be a precipitous fall in the plasma potassium due to dilution of extracellular potassium by administration of intravenous fluids, the movement of potassium into cells as a result of treatment with insulin, and the continuing renal loss of this ion.

The severity of the ketoacidosis can be assessed rapidly by measuring the plasma bicarbonate; <12 mmol/l indicates severe acidosis. The hydrogen ion concentration in the blood gives an even more precise measure but it may not be so readily available. There is no simple and accurate quantitative method for the determination of ketones in plasma although a test-strip (Ketostix) can be used as a semi-quantitative guide to the acetoacetate and acetone concentration.

Treatment

Diabetic ketoacidosis is a medical emergency which should be treated with urgency in hospital. The state of consciousness is very variable and a patient with dangerous ketosis requiring urgent treatment may walk into hospital. For this reason the term 'diabetic ketoacidosis' is to be preferred to the commonly used designation, 'diabetic coma', which suggests that there is no urgency until unconsciousness occurs. Intravenous therapy is required since, even when the patient is able to swallow, fluids given by mouth may be poorly absorbed. Treatment must be checked against the plasma concentration of glucose, potassium and bicarbonate estimated at intervals of 1–2 hours initially. The components of treatment are: 1. the administration of unmodified insulin by intramuscular or intravenous injection; 2. fluid replacement; 3. potassium replacement; and 4. the administration of antibiotics if infection is present. Note that although leucocytosis is invariably seen it represents a stress response and does not necessarily indicate infection, also that pyrexia may not be present initially because of vasodilatation secondary to acidosis.

Insulin: A loading dose of 10–20 U unmodified insulin is given by intramuscular injection immediately and 4–6 U hourly thereafter, either by intramuscular injection or intravenous infusion, preferably using a constant rate pump. The blood glucose concentration should fall by 3–6 mmol/l/h. If there is no fall in the blood glucose concentration by two hours after treatment, then the dose of insulin should be doubled until a satisfactory response is obtained. When the blood glucose concentration has fallen to 10.0 mmol/l the dose of insulin should be reduced to 1–4 U hourly.

Fluid replacement: The deficit of extracellular fluid should be made good by infusion of isotonic saline (0.9% NaCl). Early, rapid rehydration is essential otherwise the administered insulin will not reach the poorly perfused tissues. In cases which are severely acidotic (pH < 7.0), 500 ml of the isotonic saline may be replaced by isotonic sodium bicarbonate (1.4%). Correction of the total bicarbonate deficit should not be attempted, however, since there is some evidence that rapid correction of acidosis may aggravate tissue hypoxia and also reduce the level of consciousness by causing a paradoxical acidosis of cerebral spinal fluid. The combined administration of bicarbonate and insulin will also increase the risk of hypokalaemia and potassium should be given along with bicarbonate.

The intracellular deficit of water must be replaced by using 5 or 10% dextrose and not by more saline. It is

best given when the blood glucose concentration is approaching normal.

Potassium: As the plasma potassium is often high at presentation treatment with intravenous potassium chloride should be started cautiously (not more than 20 mmol/hr) and carefully monitored by frequent estimations. Sufficient should be given to maintain a normal plasma concentration and large amounts may be required (100–300 mmol in the first 24 hours).

Antibiotics: Infections must be carefully sought and vigorously treated since it may not be possible to abolish ketosis until they are controlled.

Treatment of *hyperosmolar non-ketotic diabetic coma* differs from that of ketoacidotic coma in two main respects. Firstly, these patients seem to be relatively sensitive to insulin and approximately half the dose of insulin should usually be employed. Secondly, the plasma osmolality should be measured or (less accurately) calculated (using the formula $2 \times$ sodium [mosmol/l] + $2 \times$ potassium [mosmol/l] + glucose [mosmol/l] + urea [mosmol/l] = 280–300 mosmol/l normally) and if it is high (> 360 mosmol/l) 0.45% saline should be given until the osmolality approaches normal, when 0.9% should be substituted. The rate of fluid replacement should be regulated on the basis of the central venous pressure, and plasma sodium concentration should also be checked frequently. Too rapid a fall in osmolality may be associated with the development of cerebral oedema.

In coma due to *lactic acidosis* the patient is likely to be a diabetic taking a biguanide who is very ill and overbreathing but not so profoundly dehydrated as is usual in coma due to ketoacidosis and whose breath does not smell of acetone. Ketonuria is mild or even absent yet the plasma bicarbonate and pH are markedly reduced (pH < 7.2). The diagnosis is confirmed by a high (usually > 5.0 mosmol/l) concentration of lactic acid in the blood. Treatment is with large amounts of intravenous bicarbonate as well as insulin and glucose. Despite energetic treatment the mortality in this condition is greater than 50%.

RESULTS OF TREATMENT

The long-term results of treatment of diabetes are

Table 8.19

Approximate Figures for Causes of Deaths in Treated Diabetic Patients

Atherosclerosis	70%
Renal failure	10%
Cancer	10%
Infections	6%
Diabetic ketoacidosis	1%
Other	3%

disappointing in many patients. Although few now die in diabetic keotacidosis (Table 8.19), treated diabetic patients incur an overall mortality $2\frac{1}{2}$ times greater than in a comparable non-diabetic population (Table 8.20), and also experience substantial morbidity due to vascular disease affecting both large and small blood vessels.

Large blood vessel disease accounts for about 70% of all deaths. Atherosclerosis occurs commonly and extensively in diabetic patients, with pathological changes similar to those seen in non-diabetics but occurring earlier and being more widespread.

The disease of small blood vessels is specific to diabetes and is termed *diabetic microangiopathy*. It contributes to the mortality, particularly that incurred by younger people, by causing renal failure due to *diabetic nephropathy*, and is responsible for serious disability in some patients, including blindness or severely impaired vision due to *diabetic retinopathy* as

Table 8.20

Mortality Ratios for Diabetics and Matched Controls

		Significance of increased ratio seen in diabetics
Overall	2.6	$P < 0.001$
Coronary heart disease Cerebrovascular disease Peripheral vascular disease	2.8	$P < 0.001$
All other causes including renal failure	2.7	$P < 0.05$

(Data of Pell and D'Alonzo, 1970)

well as difficulty in walking, chronic ulceration of the feet, and bowel and bladder dysfunction due to *diabetic neuropathy*. Many of these patients will also of course be disabled by the effects of atherosclerosis, such as angina, cardiac failure, intermittent claudication and gangrene.

Aetiology of Diabetic Microangiopathy

It appears that the vascular disease is secondary to the metabolic abnormalities occurring in diabetes since it is found in both primary and secondary diabetes and can be produced experimentally in animals rendered diabetic by various methods. Moreover data from clinical studies strongly suggest that although genetic factors may affect the susceptibility to develop complications, the incidence of the clinical syndromes arising from the generalised microangiopathy, i.e. retinopathy, nephropathy and neuropathy, are related to the degree of metabolic control achieved (Fig. 8.45). Whether this is due to hyperglycaemia *per se* or to some other metabolic manifestation of diabetes is unknown. Several different processes may be involved, including

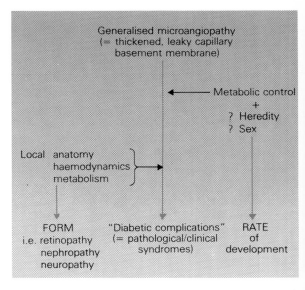

Fig. 8.45 *The evolution of diabetic complications. The main factors related to their development are duration of diabetes and the degree of metabolic control achieved.*

Table 8.21

*Possible Biochemical Causes of the
Long-term Complications of Diabetes*

Microangiopathy
    Protein glycosylation
    Increased basement membrane synthesis

Neuropathy
    Increased sorbitol synthesis
    Decreased myo-inositol levels
    Protein glycosylation

Macroangiopathy
    Increased lipid levels/synthesis
    Hyperinsulinaemia

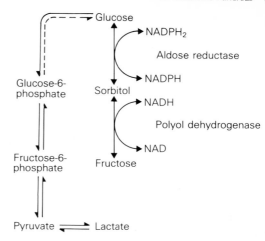

Fig. 8.46 *The polyol pathway.*

protein glycosylation, enhanced basement membrane synthesis, disturbed polyol metabolism and hyperinsulinaemia (Table. 8.21).

Biochemical Basis of the Complications of Diabetes

Protein glycosylation

Glycosylated proteins almost certainly have altered physical properties, and it is a strong possibility that such changes may be related to at least some of the long-term manifestations of poorly controlled diabetes.

Increased basement membrane synthesis

Thickening of the basement membrane of the capillaries is the hallmark of diabetic microangiopathy. It is generally considered that increased synthesis rather than decreased degradation occurs. Basement membrane consists of a collagen-like glycoprotein containing complex polysaccharides and a glucosyl–galactosyl disaccharide linked to the protein chain. The disaccharide is attached through hydroxylysine. Both the hydroxylation and the glycosylation are enzymatic post-translational processes. Analysis of glomerular basement membrane from diabetics shows increased hydroxylysine and disaccharide units with increased activity of the glycosyl transferase. There is also an increase in total basement membrane material.

Changes in polyol metabolism

An increase in sorbitol content accompanies high-glucose levels in many tissues due to the non-rate-limiting nature of the enzyme aldose reductase (Fig. 8.46). Although high sorbitol content of diabetic nerve probably does not cause osmotic disruption, inhibition of aldose reductase does cause some slight improvement in motor nerve conduction velocity in both man and experimental animals. The mechanism remains obscure.

Changes in myo-inositol metabolism

The concentration of myo-inositol is low in nerves obtained from diabetic subjects. Myo-inositol plays a critical role in phospholipid synthesis (Fig. 8.47) which forms an integral part of myelin and the neuronal cell membrane. Phosphotidyl inositol is also important as an intracellular mediator of hormonal and neurotransmitter action. The mechanism for the decrease in nerve inositol is obscure but must remain as one of the putative contributors to nerve damage in diabetic patients.

Hyperinsulinaemia

The plasma insulin concentration is raised in some

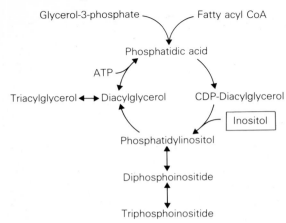

Fig. 8.47 *Metabolism of myoinositol.*

Table 8.22

Diabetic Retinopathy:
The Size of the Problem in the UK

2% diabetic = 1 000 000 diabetics
2% blind   = 20 000 blind diabetics

(Data of Cheng, 1979)

Table 8.23

The Clinical Features
Characteristic of Diabetic
Retinopathy

Microaneurysms
Retinal haemorrhages
Hard exudates
Venous dilatation
Increased tortuosity of vessels
New vessel formation
Preretinal haemorrhage
Vitreous haemorrhage
Fibrous proliferation

NIDDM patients and in all insulin-treated diabetics. In the latter this occurs because the conventional treatment involves subcutaneous injections and, to achieve normal hepatic insulinisation, excessive amounts of insulin must be given peripherally. This is very different from the normal situation, where insulin is secreted intraportally and insulinisation of the liver is easily achieved by the extraction of 50% of the insulin which reaches it so that the concentration of insulin in peripheral blood is low. It has been shown experimentally that insulin stimulates lipid synthesis in large arteries and it is possible that this accelerates the atherosclerotic process in the diabetic.

Pathophysiology and Clinical Aspects of the Long-term Complications of Diabetes

Diabetic retinopathy

Retinopathy is the commonest long-term complication of diabetes. In most cases it produces no symptoms but it can cause blindness and diabetic retinopathy is the single most common cause of blindness in Britain today, accounting for 16% of all those blind (Table 8.22). Table 8.23 lists the clinical features characteristic of diabetic retinopathy, two of which are illustrated in Fig. 8.48. However, the first pathological signs of diabetic microangiopathy in the retina, that is increased blood flow and areas of capillary closure, are not detectable clinically but may be demonstrated by fluorescein angiography (Fig. 8.49).

The metabolism of many, if not most, diabetic patients being treated by conventional methods is far from normal and numerous functional abnormalities have been identified in their blood. Potentially any one or several of these might play a role in causing diabetic microangiopathy and a concept of the development of diabetic retinopathy is illustrated in Fig. 8.50.

An extremely important area currently the subject of much controversy is the reversibility of diabetic retinopathy. Using the new methods of delivering insulin it is possible to lower the blood glucose concentration rapidly to normal (p. 194). As a result we know that in general if the body weight and the blood glucose concentration are normal all the metabolic abnormalities listed above the dotted line in Fig. 8.50 will disappear. However, the reversibility of lesions below the line is much less certain. Indeed there is some evidence that rapid reduction of a raised blood glucose

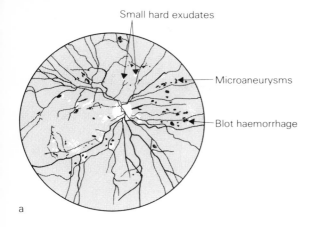

Small hard exudates

Microaneurysms

Blot haemorrhage

a

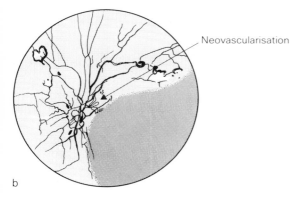

Neovascularisation

b

Fig. 8.48 *Ophthalmoscopic view of (a) simple background retinopathy with microaneurysms, small blot retinal haemorrhages, and small hard exudates, (b) proliferative retinopathy with neovascularisation arising from the optic disc and preretinal (subhyaloid) haemorrhage.*

concentration to normal might, at least initially, accelerate the progression of clinically detectable retinopathy rather than ameliorate it, possibly by diminishing retinal blood flow.

Clinical features: In most cases, *microaneurysms* are the earliest clinical abnormality detected. They appear as minute, discrete, circular, dark red spots near to but apparently separate from the retinal vessels. They look like tiny haemorrhages but photography of injected preparations of retina shows they are in fact minute aneurysms of capillaries (Fig. 8.51) mainly arising near areas of capillary closure.

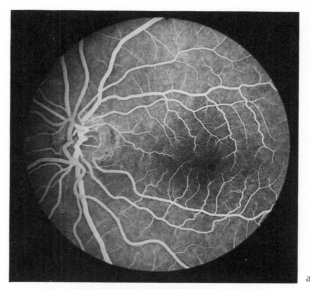

a

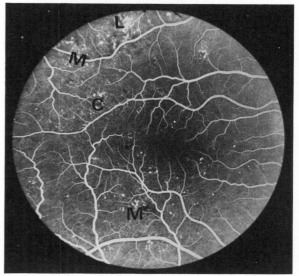

b

Fig. 8.49 *Fundus fluorescein angiogram in (a) a normal subject, (b) patient with diabetic retinopathy showing areas of capillary closure (C), numerous microaneurysms (M), and leakage from new vessel systems (L). (Courtesy Dr Eva Kohner, Hammersmith Hospital, London.)*

Haemorrhages most characteristically occur in the deeper layers of the retina and hence are round and regular in shape and described as 'blot' haemorrhages. The smaller ones may be difficult to differentiate from microaneurysms and the two are often grouped

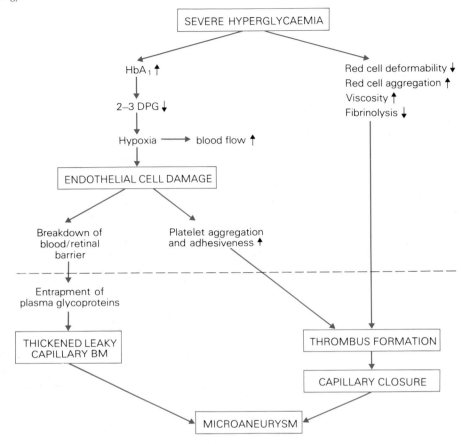

Fig. 8.50 *A concept of the development of diabetic retino-pathy. The effect of increased glycosylation of haemoglobin on oxygen delivery to the tissues is complex. 2,3-DPG is a product of red cell metabolism which tends to displace oxygen from haemoglobin. In situations where the oxygen delivery to the tissues is reduced (for example in those who are anaemic, smoke or have mild/moderate hyperglycaemia) 2,3-DPG tends to show a compensatory rise. However since 2,3-DPG occupies the same binding sites as glucose on the haemoglobin molecule, more severe glycosylation will tend to reduce binding of 2,3-DPG leading to an increase in the oxygen affinity of the haemoglobin molecule and reduced oxygen delivery to the tissues. This in turn leads to dilatation and increased permeability at the venous end of the capillary. A reduction in red cell deformability and an increase in red cell aggregation aggravate the tendency to tissue hypoxia by causing capillary occlusion.*

together and referred to as 'dot and blot' haemorrhages.

Soft exudates, similar to those seen in hypertension, occur but *hard exudates* are more common and characteristic of diabetic retinopathy. They vary in size from tiny specks to large confluent patches. They result from leakage of plasma from abnormal retinal capillaries and overlie areas of neuronal degeneration.

New vessels ('neovascularisation') may arise from mature vessels on the optic disc or the retina. The earliest appearance is that of fine tufts of delicate vessels forming arcades on the surface of the retina. As they grow they may extend forward towards the vitreous. They are fragile and leaky and are liable to rupture, causing haemorrhage which may be intra-retinal, preretinal ('subhyaloid') or into the vitreous.

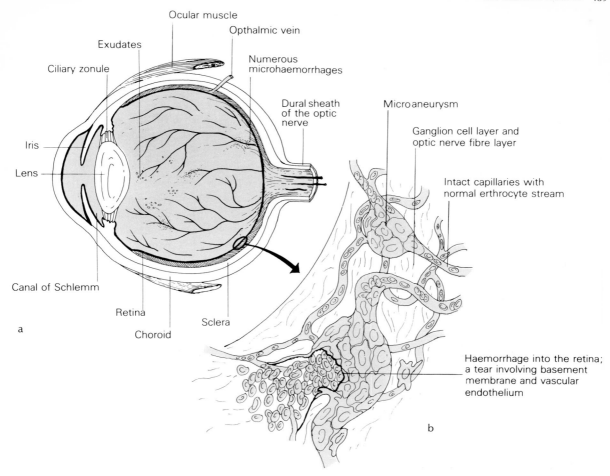

Fig. 8.51 *(a) Macrostructure of the eye, (b) microstructure of retina with microaneurysm and retinal haemorrhage.*

Serous products leaking from these new vessel systems stimulate a connective tissue reaction, *retinitis proliferans*. This first appears as a white, cloudy haze among the network of new vessels. As it extends, the new vessels may be obliterated and the surrounding retina covered by a dense white sheet. At this stage bleeding is less common but retinal detachment can occur due to contraction of adhesions between the vitreous and the retina.

Classification: A classification of diabetic retinopathy based on prognosis for vision is shown in Table 8.24. Microaneurysms, abnormalities of the veins, and small blot haemorrhages and hard exudates will not interfere seriously with vision unless they are associated with macular oedema or directly involve the macula. Unfortunately all these lesions occur most commonly in the perimacular area and as they enlarge are likely to impinge on the macula so that visual acuity is seriously impaired. New vessels may be *completely symptomless* until sudden visual loss occurs from a haemorrhage into the vitreous. Although these frequently clear, the

Table 8.24

Classification of Diabetic Retinopathy Based on Prognosis for Vision

Simple background retinopathy without maculopathy
microaneurysms
small blot retinal haemorrhages
small hard exudates

GOOD 5-YEAR PROGNOSIS

Premalignant retinopathy
hard exudates in rings or plaques
multiple soft exudates
sheets/clusters/large blot haemorrhages
venous loops and 'bleeding'

Malignant retinopathy
exudative maculopathy
preretinal haemorrhage
neovascularisation
fibrous proliferation

IF UNTREATED, 50% ARE BLIND WITHIN 5 YEARS

risk of recurrence is high and the more frequent the haemorrhage the slower and less complete the recovery. Fibrous tissue may seriously interfere with vision by obscuring the retina and/or causing retinal detachment.

Prevention and treatment: As retinopathy seems to be secondary to the metabolic abnormality and good metabolic control may reduce the chance of its development every effort should be made to maintain a normal metabolic state in all diabetic patients from the time of presentation. It is a common error to suppose that NIDDM is 'mild' and carries little risk of complications. This is not so. Whatever the type of diabetes, duration of the disorder and sustained hyperglycaemia are the main factors associated with the development of microangiopathy.

Simple retinopathy without maculopathy is not associated with significant impairment of vision and no specific treatment is indicated. Retinopathy may be aggravated by hypertension, hyperlipidaemia, smoking and excessive ingestion of alcohol, so therapeutic intervention should be directed at these.

Premalignant and malignant retinopathy can be treated with retinal photocoagulation. Photocoagulation is used, 1, to destroy areas of retinal ischaemia (since it is thought that this plays a major role in the development of neovascularisation), 2, to seal leaking microaneurysms and exudates and, 3, to obliterate new vessels directly. Two types of photocoagulation are available: xenon-arc (white light) and laser beam (monochromatic blue/green light). The latter is less uncomfortable for the patient and the smaller size of the beam allows greater accuracy in delivering shots. This procedure can be done under local anaesthesia

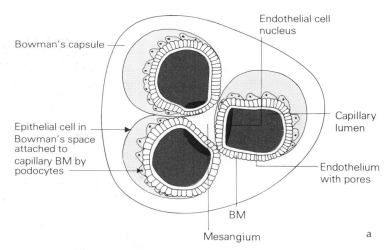

Fig. 8.52 *(a) Ultrastructure of the glomerulus: cross-section of a normal capillary lobule. (b) Microstructure of glomerulus with thickened basement membrane.*

and in skilled, experienced hands is a simple procedure which carries little risk and can be very effective.

Because diabetic retinopathy is now a treatable condition if diagnosed early, *when it is commonly symptomless,* all diabetic patients must have their eyes examined regularly by a competent observer using a mydriatic to obtain adequate visualisation of the retina. Once there is evidence of progression of simple retinopathy, and particularly whenever new vessels are seen, patients must be referred to an ophthalmologist for further supervision and treatment.

Diabetic nephropathy

The earliest renal change detected in diabetic patients is glomerular hyper-perfusion. This is followed by renal hypertrophy. At this stage there may be microalbuminuria which is reversible by strict control of the blood glucose concentration. Its importance is that it predicts the development of irreversible renal damage if treatment of diabetes is not intensified. Later a specific type of renal lesion may occur as a result of thickening of the basement membrane of the glomerular capillaries. The ultrastructure of the normal glomerulus is shown in Fig. 8.52 (a) and the evolution of diabetic nephropathy in Fig. 8.53. Pathologically there are two types of diabetic glomerular sclerosis: diffuse and nodular. The former is more common and consists of a generalised thickening of the basement membrane. The nodular type is a development of this, in which rounded masses

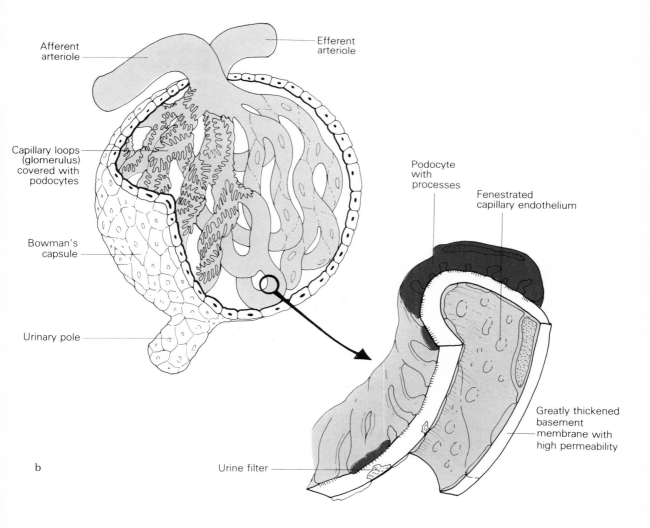

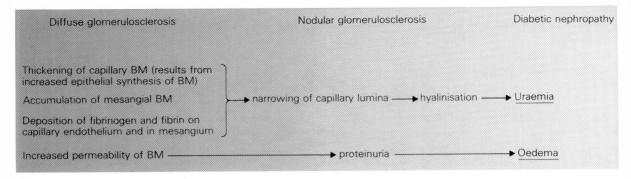

Fig. 8.53 *Development of diabetic renal disease.*

of hyaline material (sometimes called Kimmelstiel-Wilson bodies) are superimposed upon the diffuse lesions (Fig. 8.53).

Even in well-established diabetic glomerular sclerosis the patient may exhibit only slight to moderate proteinuria. In some instances, however, marked proteinuria and the nephrotic syndrome develop, with increasing renal failure and uraemia.

Treatment: There is some evidence that improved metabolic control can reverse and delay the progression of early diabetic nephropathy and that the treatment of hypertension will contribute to this. In the later stages the condition becomes irreversible and the management is the same as in other forms of chronic renal disease, though results of haemodialysis are less good than in non-diabetics. The place of long-term continuous ambulatory peritoneal dialysis (CAPD) is uncertain but seems promising. The results of renal transplantation in carefully selected cases can be almost as good as in non-diabetics and use of cyclos-

porin has improved results in non-diabetic and diabetic alike. Unfortunately many diabetics will not qualify for active intervention because of other disabilities such as severe large blood vessel disease, neuropathy and retinopathy.

Diabetic neuropathy

Neuropathy is an early and common complication in diabetic patients. It is symptomless in the majority of patients but causes severe disability in a few. In those with clinically apparent autonomic neuropathy, the five-year mortality is 50%. Like retinopathy, it occurs secondary to the metabolic disturbance and the prevalence of neuropathy is related to the duration of diabetes and the degree of metabolic control.

Pathophysiology: The structural components of myelinated nerve fibres and the pathological features of diabetic neuropathy are shown in Fig. 8.54. Abnormalities of the intraneural capillaries, i.e. thickening of the basement membrane and microthrombi, are also seen.

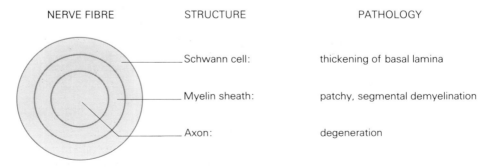

Fig. 8.54 *Diabetic neuropathy: histopathology.*

Classification: Various classifications of diabetic neuropathy have been proposed, one of which is shown in Table 8.25. None of the proposed classifications is entirely satisfactory since motor, sensory and autonomic nerves may be involved in varying combinations so that clinically mixed syndromes frequently occur.

Clinical features: Symmetrical sensory polyneuropathy is frequently asymptomatic. Signs found on physical examination commonly include loss of tendon reflexes in the lower limbs, diminished perception of vibration sensation distally, and 'glove and stocking' impairment of all modalities of sensation. Symptoms include parasthesiae in the feet and sometimes in the hands, pain in the lower limbs (dull, aching and/or lancinating and worse at night), burning sensations in the soles of the feet, cutaneous hyperaesthesia and difficulty in walking. There may be perforating and chronic ulcers in the feet and painless distal arthropathy (Charcot's joints). There may also be some motor involvement causing muscle weakness and wasting. On investigation both motor and sensory conduction velocity are reduced.

Symptomatic relief and a degree of functional improvement can be achieved by normalising the blood glucose concentration (e.g. by a continuous infusion of insulin, p. 194). The administration of aldose reductase inhibitors may also be useful.

Mononeuropathy: Either motor or sensory function can be affected within a single peripheral or cranial nerve. The nerves most commonly affected are the third and sixth cranial nerves resulting in diplopia due to impaired ocular movement; the ulnar and median nerves leading to the clinical picture of carpal tunnel compression syndrome; and the femoral, sciatic and lateral popliteal nerves leading to foot drop. Local vascular occlusion may be particularly important in the aetiology of mononeuropathy and entrapment syndromes.

Diabetic amyotrophy is an asymmetrical motor neuropathy presenting as severe progressive weakness and wasting of the proximal muscles of the lower (and occasionally also the upper) limbs and commonly accompanied by severe pain. Sometimes there may also be marked loss of weight ('neuropathic cachexia'). With intensive insulin treatment the prognosis is good and most patients recover over a period of months or years.

Autonomic neuropathy is not necessarily associated with peripheral somatic neuropathy. Either parasympathetic or sympathetic fibres or both may be affected in any one or more systems in an individual patient, and the symptoms and signs vary from one patient to another.

In the *cardiovascular system*, postural hypotension may occur as a result of damage to the sympathetic vasoconstrictor supply to arteries in the lower limbs and splanchnic bed. There may also be resting tachycardia and loss of heart rate variation on deep breathing and standing up from the horizontal position.

In the *gastrointestinal* tract there may be oesophageal atony, gastroparesis and nocturnal diarrhoea with faecal incontinence.

Genitourinary autonomic neuropathy commonly causes impotence and may also result in an atonic bladder with recurrent urinary tract infection and overflow incontinence.

Sudomotor phenomena include 'gustatory sweating', i.e. profuse perspiration of the head and neck following ingestion of cheese or curry; drenching nocturnal sweats; and anhidrosis leading to fissures in the feet.

Vasomotor phenomena include loss of skin vasomotor responses (patients complain of constantly cold feet) and dependent oedema due to loss of vasomotor tone and increased vascular permeability.

Pupillary abnormalities commonly seen include de-

Table 8.25

Classification of Diabetic Neuropathy

Somatic
1. Symmetrical, mainly sensory, polyneuropathy
   chronic
   acute
2. Mononeuropathy (mononeuropathy multiplex)
3. Asymmetrical, mainly motor, polyneuropathy
   ('Diabetic amyotrophy')

Visceral (autonomic)
   cardiovascular
   gastrointestinal
   genitourinary
   sudomotor
   vasomotor
   pupillary
   loss of awareness of hypoglycaemia

creased pupil size, resistance to mydriatics and delayed or absent response to light.

Loss of awareness of hypoglycaemia due to sympathetic neuropathy is common in long-standing diabetes (see p. 181).

The development of autonomic neuropathy is less clearly related to poor metabolic control than somatic neuropathy, and impoved control rarely results in amelioration of symptoms.

Diabetes in Pregnancy

Pregnancy in diabetic women is associated with an increased perinatal mortality rate, either from stillbirth due to sudden intrauterine death in pregnancy or neonatal death due to the respiratory distress syndrome and/or congenital malformation. Birth trauma is also more common, due to excessively large babies. All these problems are directly related to poor metabolic control and largely disappear if normoglycaemia is maintained in the mother before and at the time of conception and throughout pregnancy.

Prospects in Diabetes Mellitus

Treatment

The scale of the clinical problem presented by patients with microangiopathy, the suggestion that good control of blood glucose may prevent or retard the development of diabetic complications, the introduction of better methods of assessing diabetic control, the realisation that at present good control is achieved in only a minority of diabetic patients, and increased understanding of the deficiencies of conventional treatment has led to a search for better methods of treatment (Table 8.26). 'Open loop' systems are battery-powered portable pumps providing continuous subcutaneous, intramuscular or intravenous infusion of insulin, delivered at fixed rates (a low basal rate and one or more higher rates before main meals) without reference to the blood glucose concentration. In practice the 'loop' is closed by the patient performing blood glucose estimations and the use of these devices requires a high degree of patient motivation and has the particular disadvantage that if the pump fails the

---

Table 8.26

New Systems for Delivering Insulin

'Open loop'
'Closed loop'
Pancreatic transplantation
Islet transplantation

---

onset of ketosis tends to be more rapid than with conventional treatment because there is no subcutaneous depot of insulin. These systems will not be suitable for general therapeutic use until they incorporate an automatic failure alarm and a miniaturised glucose sensor. The latter is not yet available.

'Closed loop', sometimes referred to as 'artificial pancreas' systems will consist of three basic components: a glucose sensor, an insulin delivery pump and a computer control which regulates the administration of insulin on the basis of the blood glucose concentration. Ideally such a device should be small enough for implantation, deliver insulin intraportally, and measure the blood glucose rapidly without consuming blood. Existing systems deliver insulin peripherally, use blood, and are large, extracorporeal, relatively slow and unreliable and very expensive. However, technology is advancing rapidly, particularly in relation to miniaturisation and glucose sensor devices.

Pancreatic transplantation is still at an early phase of development and at present is reserved for those patients in the highest risk categories whose prognosis is poor.

Transplantation of isolated pancreatic islets into the splenic capsule has been successful in animals. Although in man there are major problems in relation to both the supply of islets and their rejection following transplantation, this may prove to be a more satisfactory approach in the long run.

Prevention

From a public health standpoint the only cost-effective way of dealing with diabetes is to prevent it.

NIDDM is a disease of the prosperous and is associated with an affluent lifestyle. NIDDM is likely to arise in genetically predisposed persons who eat too much and exercise too little. Effective health education of the population could reduce the incidence of clinically expressed disease, while screening for diabetes (particularly in high-risk groups), and more vigorous and early treatment of NIDDM would reduce the incidence of serious vascular disease in these patients.

The fact that islet B cells are destroyed slowly over several years before clinical presentation offers the hope that, in the future, it might be possible to identify prediabetic insulin-dependent patients (by, e.g., such techniques as HLA typing combined with measurement of immunological indices), to protect their viable pancreatic B cells from further damage by immunological manipulation, and perhaps even to induce them to regenerate.

SPONTANEOUS HYPOGLYCAEMIA

Normally, a finely tuned balance exists between the flow of glucose into and out of the glucose pool (p. 151), and the blood glucose concentration is maintained remarkably constant in the range 2.5–7.5 mmol/l at all times.

Hypoglycaemia, defined as a blood glucose concentration of 2.2 mmol/l or less, is always pathological, but those whose random blood glucose concentration lies within the range 2.2–2.5 mmol/l form a heterogeneous group which includes some individuals at one end of the normal distribution curve.

Hypoglycaemia results from either increased removal of glucose from, or reduced entry of glucose into, the pool, or from a combination of both mechanisms.

Classification

There are many causes of hypoglycaemia. The main factors affecting glucose homeostasis are gastric emptying and intestinal absorption, hepatic production of glucose, and the secretion of insulin and the counter-regulatory hormones. In Table 8.27, the causes of hypoglycaemia are, for convenience, grouped under these headings.

Table 8.27

Classification of Hypoglycaemia

Reactive hypoglycaemia
  induced by:
    glucose: postgastrectomy
               peptic ulceration hypermotility
               early diabetes
               'idiopathic'
    galactose: galactosaemia
    fructose: hereditary fructose intolerance
    leucine: leucine hypersensitivity

Hepatic disease
  hepatocellular
  congestive cardiac failure
  neoplastic
  glycogen storage disease
  defective gluconeogenesis:
    alcohol-induced
    pyruvate carboxylase deficiency

Inappropriate insulin secretion
  insulin-secreting tumour:
    benign
    malignant
    microadenomatosis
  islet hyperplasia
  pluriglandular syndrome
  nesidioblastosis
  neonatal hypoglycaemia:
    infants of diabetic mothers
    erythroblastosis fetalis

Counter-regulatory hormone insufficiency
  pituitary
  adrenocortical
  thyroid
  catecholamines ⎱ in long-standing insulin-dependent
  glucagon   ⎰ diabetic patients

Miscellaneous
  extrapancreatic neoplasms – particularly mesenchymal
  drug-induced:
    salicylates
    beta blockers
    sulphonylureas
    insulin:
      inadvertent
      factitious
  starvation
  prolonged exercise
  end-stage renal disease
  autoimmune insulin syndrome

Note—By far the most common cause of severe hypoglycaemia is insulin treatment for diabetes. Treatment with sulphonylurea drugs is the next most common cause, followed by glucose-induced reactive hypoglycaemia and factitious hypoglycaemia. All other causes are rare.

Diagnosis

The diagnosis depends on the demonstration of a venous true blood glucose concentration of < 2.5 mmol/l. It is essential that particular care is taken in relation to both the collection of blood samples and the method of estimating the blood glucose concentration. Venous blood samples should be placed immediately in a tube containing a substance to inhibit glycolysis (e.g. sodium fluoride or iodoacetate) and then refrigerated until analysis, which should be performed within 24 hours. Alternatively, a heparinised sample can be collected and the plasma separated and frozen immediately. A sensitive, accurate and specific (i.e. enzymatic) method must be used to estimate the blood glucose concentration. It should be remembered that the plasma glucose concentration is 15% higher than that for whole blood (p. 159).

The ideal time to collect a blood sample for glucose measurement in cases where hypoglycaemia is suspected is at an early stage during a hypoglycaemic attack. The symptoms of hypoglycaemia are described on p. 180. However, hypoglycaemia is not always accompanied by symptoms and, in these circumstances, samples of blood should be obtained on several occasions after an overnight fast and also 4–5 hours after food.

Once hypoglycaemia has been documented, the cause must be identified. When gastric, hepatic and renal disease, inborn errors of metabolism, endocrine disorders, drugs which might induce hypoglycaemia, and extrapancreatic tumours have been excluded, the diagnostic problem consists of distinguishing between glucose-induced reactive hypoglycaemia, an insulin-secreting lesion, and factitious hypoglycaemia. Dynamic function tests are employed to clarify this.

In an extended oral glucose tolerance test, samples of blood are obtained before, and at half-hourly intervals after, 50 g glucose orally for at least 5 hours for estimation of plasma glucose and immunoreactive insulin concentration. In normal individuals, plasma glucose and insulin are closely related (Fig. 8.9) while in patients with hypoglycaemia they are asynchronous with an inappropriately high plasma insulin concentration at some stage in the test. Characteristic patterns of plasma glucose and insulin are seen in the various types of hypoglycaemia (Fig. 8.55).

In the C-peptide suppression test, unmodified insulin

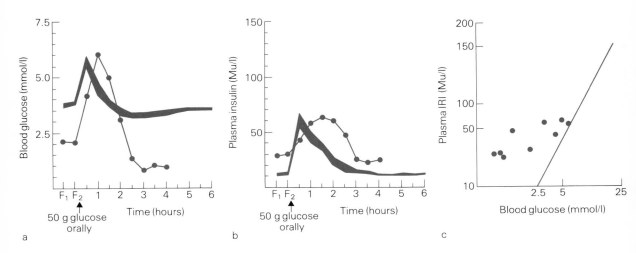

Fig. 8.55 *Extended glucose tolerance test in a patient with an insulinoma showing fasting and postabsorptive hypoglycaemia (a) with associated hyperinsulinaemia (b). (The thick red line represents the mean ± SEM values for normal subjects.) The loss of synchrony between the blood glucose and plasma insulin concentrations is more clearly seen when they are plotted against each other as in (c). The diagonal line represents the normal exponential relationship with the plasma IRI undetectable below the lower limit of the assay (in this case 10 Mu/l) when the blood glucose falls to < 2.5 mmol/l. The insulinoma patient has measurable circulating insulin when the blood glucose concentration is < 2.5 mmol/l.*

is administered in a dosage of 0.1 units/kg body weight, to a maximum of 10 units; blood samples are obtained at 15-minute intervals thereafter for 2 hours for measurement of plasma glucose and C-peptide concentration. Provided the venous blood glucose concentration falls to < 2.2 mmol/l, in normal subjects and in patients with reactive hypoglycaemia plasma C-peptide is suppressed to an undetectable level. In contrast, plasma C-peptide is not suppressed in patients with an insulin-secreting tumour. This test has largely replaced the tedious and expensive prolonged (72 hours) fast previously used for this purpose.

If these tests suggest an insulin-secreting tumour then further investigation is indicated to try to: 1. obtain evidence of malignancy; 2. exclude the pluriglandular syndrome; and 3. locate the tumour. The latter may be difficult since insulinomas are commonly very small (frequently < 1 cm). Scanning by computerised axial tomography, coeliac axis arteriography and transhepatic venous blood sampling for C-peptide and immunoreactive insulin measurements may be helpful.

Treatment

The vast majority of cases of reactive hypoglycaemia respond well to dietary measures consisting of exclusion of sucrose and frequent and regular meals high in fibre.

Insulinomas should be removed surgically but, if it is impossible to locate the tumour, treatment with diazoxide, sometimes combined with chlorothiazide, is very effective in many cases and the side-effects are few. These drugs inhibit the release of insulin from the pancreatic beta cell. Streptozotocin is used in the treatment of neoplastic insulin-secreting tumours. This also is very effective, but the margin between the therapeutic and toxic dose is narrow. Somatostatin (or rather, the synthetic, specifically insulin-inhibitory, prolonged-action analogues of somatostatin) may also prove to be valuable.

Further Reading

Anderson D.C., Winter J.S.D. (eds.) (1985). *Adrenal Cortex*. London: Butterworth.

Beardwell C., Robertson G.L. (1981). *The Pituitary*. London: Butterworth.

Belchetz P.E. (1984). *Management of Pituitary Disease*. London: Chapman & Hall Medical.

Black P.McL., Zervas N.T., Ridgway E.C., Martin J.B. (1984). *Secretory tumours of the pituitary gland. Progress in Endocrine Research and Therapy Vol. I*. New York: Raven Press.

Gray C.H., James V.H.T. (1983). *Hormones in Blood* Vol. 5, 3rd edn. London: Academic Press.

Hall R., Anderson J., Smart G.A., Besser G.M. (1982). *The Fundamentals of Clinical Endocrinology*, 3rd edn. London: Pitman.

Heath D.A., Marx S.J. (1982). *Calcium Disorders*. London: Butterworth.

James V.H.T. (ed.) (1979). The adrenal gland. In *Comprehensive Endocrinology*. New York: Raven Press.

James W.P.T. (ed.) (1984). Obesity. In *Clinics in Endocrinology and Metabolism*, Vol. 13/No. 3. London: W. B. Saunders Company.

Jocelyn E.P. (1985). *Diabetes Mellitus*. Philadelphia: Lea & Febiger.

Ney R.L. (ed.) (1985). Investigations of endocrine disorders. In *Clinics in Endocrinology and Metabolism*, Vol. 14/No. 1. London: W. B. Saunders Company.

Olefsky J.M., Sherwin R.S. (1985). *Diabetes Mellitus: Management and Complications*. New York and Edinburgh: Churchill Livingstone.

Scanlon M.F. (ed.) (1983). Neuroendocrinology. In *Clinics in Endocrinology and Metabolism*, Vol. 12/No. 3. London: W. B. Saunders Company.

Toft A.D. (ed.) (1985). Hyperthyroidism. In *Clinics in Endocrinology and Metabolism*, Vol. 14/No. 2. London: W. B. Saunders Company.

Wilson J.D., Foster D.W. (eds.) (1985). *Williams' Textbook of Endocrinology*, 7th edn. Philadelphia: W. B. Saunders Company.

Index